FLUENT APHASIA

Fluent aphasia is a language disorder that follows brain damage, causing difficulty in finding the correct words and in structuring sentences. Speakers also experience problems in understanding language, and this severely impairs their ability to communicate. In this informative and up-to-date study, Susan Edwards provides a detailed description of fluent aphasia, by drawing widely on research data, and by comparing fluent aphasia with other types of aphasia, as well as with normal language. She discusses evidence that the condition affects access to underlying grammatical rules as well as to the lexicon and explores the relationship between language and the brain, the controversy over aphasia syndromes, the assessment of aphasia via standardised tests and the analysis of continuous speech data. Extensive examples of aphasic speech are given, and the progress of one fluent aphasic speaker is discussed in detail. Written by an internationally renowned expert, this book will be of interest to linguists and practitioners alike.

SUSAN EDWARDS is Professor and Head of Clinical Linguistics at the School of Linguistics and Applied Language Studies, University of Reading. She has previously published *Language and Mental Handicap* (with Jean Rondal, 1997), and is co-author of *The Reynell Developmental Scales III* (a language test used in the diagnosis and treatment of children with language disorders), and *The Verb and Sentence Test* (a clinical research tool for use with aphasia). She has also published many articles and book chapters about aphasia and other speech and language disorders.

In this series

CAMBRIDGE STUDIES IN LINGUISTICS

General editors: P. AUSTIN, J. BRESNAN, B. COMRIE,
S. CRAIN, W. DRESSLER, C. J. EWEN, R. LASS,
D. LIGHTFOOT, K. RICE, I. ROBERTS, S. ROMAINE,
N. V. SMITH

Fluent Aphasia

FLUENT APHASIA

SUSAN EDWARDS

School of Linguistics and Applied Language Studies
University of Reading

and

College of Sciences
University of Limerick

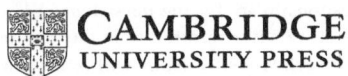

CAMBRIDGE
UNIVERSITY PRESS

CAMBRIDGE UNIVERSITY PRESS
Cambridge, New York, Melbourne, Madrid, Cape Town, Singapore, São Paulo, Delhi

Cambridge University Press
The Edinburgh Building, Cambridge CB2 8RU, UK

Published in the United States of America by Cambridge University Press, New York

www.cambridge.org
Information on this title: www.cambridge.org/9780521107495

First published 2005
This digitally printed version 2009

A catalogue record for this publication is available from the British Library

ISBN 978-0-521-79107-6 hardback
ISBN 978-0-521-10749-5 paperback

Contents

Figures

Tables

Acknowledgements

I have been privileged to study and work with many inspirational colleagues who
have contributed to the development of my ideas about language and aphasia.
I am grateful to each one although I will list only a few here. Many years ago
when I was a student, Margaret Greene, who was then a lecturer at the Central
School of Speech and Drama, London, introduced me to the study of aphasia.
She persuaded me of the need for intellectual investigation of the condition
and encouraged me to challenge accepted views. I have often thought about
the things she, as a clinician, observed about aphasia. Roelien Bastiaanse, Jane
Maxim and Cindy Thompson have, by shared discussions, debates, dinners and
drinks over a number of years, helped me form some of the ideas I try to convey
in this book. I want to thank them for sharing their intellectual vigour and their
enthusiasm for the study of language and aphasia with me, for disagreeing
with some of my ideas but especially for their personal generosity in so many
spheres of my life. I acknowledge learning from my research students, past
and present, especially Marina Arabatzi, Clare McCann, Christos Salis and
Kate Tucker. Thanks are owed to the doctoral and post-doctoral researchers in
Cindy's laboratory, and to those of my students and colleagues at the Universities
of Reading and Limerick who have, through discussion and debate, enriched
my life. Special thanks to Miseon Lee who read the whole manuscript and
helped me with the linguistic points I try to make. Any remaining errors are, of
course, mine. I am grateful to friends and colleagues who have read all or part
of this manuscript and pointed out errors. I have gained much from working
with my linguistic colleagues at the Universities of Reading and Gronigen and
elsewhere, and thank those who have taken time to try to enlighten me about
the mysteries of language. It has been fun working with so many smart people
in different universities and clinics. Thanks are due to the anonymous reviewer
who provided me with some helpful comments as well as encouragement to
finish this project. I am also grateful to Jacqueline French and Elizabeth Davey
at CUP for their considerable help in preparing the manuscript.

Finally, I would like to thank MG and his wife, who have been a delight to know, who have given generously of their time for my study and teaching of aphasia and from whom I have learnt so much. Without knowing you both, this book and my understanding of aphasia would be so much the poorer.

Introduction

Fluent aphasia is an interesting condition for various reasons. For a number of years, the existence of two types of aphasia that not only sound different but arise from different loci of cerebral damage has been used to support the notion of two independent domains of language, the grammar and the lexicon. Damage to cerebral tissue in the pre-Rolandic areas of the cortex is associated with damage to the grammar or to the computational aspects of language, while the mental lexicon, our vocabulary store, is spared. In fact it is not clear whether aphasia causes loss or damaged access to this domain of language, as we will discuss below. In contrast to this state, damage to the post-Rolandic area results in damage to the mental lexicon or access to that lexicon: the grammar, or access to the computational aspects of language, is assumed to be spared. So, these two pathological conditions that we will refer to as non-fluent and fluent aphasia, epitomise damaged grammar versus damaged lexis. To take idealised cases, non-fluent speakers exhibit grammatical errors whereas fluent aphasic speakers struggle with lexical recall. Of course, this can be seen as a gross over-simplification and we will examine the flaws in this description as we progress through the monograph, but it not only provides a good starting point but also encapsulates issues that will be explored.

This monograph is about fluent aphasia, a type of aphasia that is commonly seen in clinics but about which little is written. We will consider the language abilities of people with fluent aphasia, concentrating on their lexical and grammatical abilities. All aphasia textbooks contain descriptions of fluent aphasia (under various classifications) largely based on clinical observations rather than on empirical work. In the course of this monograph we will review various accounts of fluent aphasia. I aim, by drawing on connected speech data, to expand on the current descriptions and accounts that we have of fluent aphasic speech, concentrating on the language produced. I will discuss grammatical and lexical abilities revealed in these data and see how far lexical retrieval problems disrupt sentence structure. I will re-examine the claims that syntax remains intact. To this end, it will be necessary first to pull together available

1

descriptions, speculations and explanations of fluent aphasia. This information must then be viewed within the two contexts, of abnormal and normal language. Comparisons with abnormal language, aphasia, will focus on descriptions and explanations of non-fluent aphasia and, specifically, agrammatism. Comparisons of the features of these two types of aphasia include consideration of the explanations of agrammatism, especially explanations couched within the framework of Universal Grammar.

There are various perspectives from which fluent aphasia may be viewed. Aphasia is a condition that arises subsequent to brain damage and, as a result, changes occur to non-verbal as well as to verbal behaviour. Other consequences of brain damage may include impaired visual skills, spatial skills, memory and so on. Deficits of this nature impact on patients' ability to cope with aphasia, their ability to co-operate with testing and their chances of successful rehabilitation and, as a result, some aphasiologists and clinicians consider these behavioural deficits to be part and parcel of aphasia. I will not be taking this approach. This account focuses on the spoken output in fluent aphasia, although one chapter is devoted to the comprehension deficit, a characteristic of fluent aphasia.

Material in this monograph has been gleaned from many sources. I cite and discuss empirical research but I aim to cover or, at least, introduce the reader to various perspectives of study, including the use of continuous speech data. I have tried to give a broad view although I am aware that my selection will not be to everyone's liking. I have also tried to go beyond data and to give a flavour of how fluent aphasia touches and changes peoples' lives. The anecdotes I tell are based on my clinical experiences as a speech and language therapist and I hope they give some humanity to this study. I have learnt much from discussions I have had with other aphasiologists, not only speech and language therapists, but also neurologists, psychologists and, occasionally, some exceptional linguists. The study of aphasia seems to attract more psychologists than linguists, and linguistic analyses and linguistically motivated theories of aphasia are few and far between. I remain convinced, however, that there are rich data here for linguists to pick over.

This monograph does not adhere to any one school of aphasiology or any one theory within linguistic science: I write as a research speech and language therapist and for readers from a number of different disciplines. From time to time, I call upon theoretical linguistic notions but, in common with my fellow aphasiologists, do not follow or develop any one particular theory. I am writing for students of aphasia, whether based in psychology, linguistics, health studies, medicine or speech and language pathology. By students, I include anyone who wishes to learn about the topic, regardless of their formal level of study. I hope that readers who come from a linguistics or psychology background will gain some insights into fluent aphasia that include the person as well as the data. For those readers who come from a clinical background, I hope that my linguistic descriptions will encourage them to think about aphasic data within some linguistic framework. There will be parts of the book that may be rather technical for some readers and some that will be too basic for others. It should be possible to turn the pages or go to the next chapter and pick up the story again or select the chapters of interest. I hope that this monograph will not only give a picture of what fluent aphasia sounds like but also help the reader to understand a little about what a person with fluent aphasia experiences.

Chapter 1 starts by giving a short, general introduction to three topics: the description of fluent aphasic speech, the notion of aphasia syndromes, and the relationship between brain and language. I start by outlining the commonly recognised syndromes of aphasia. I then proceed to consider the original accounts of the disorder given by Wernicke in the nineteenth century and then move on to probably the most influential account of fluent aphasia given in the twentieth century, that by Harold Goodglass. Goodglass and his associates have been staunch advocates of the syndromic approach in aphasia research. That is, they hold that aphasia is not a unitary condition but comprises different types of aphasia and that these types constitute syndromes. While recognising the importance of syndromes, especially in aphasia research, we encounter and discuss some problems of this approach. This leads us to a short review of language-brain relationships.

In chapter 2, I extend the descriptions of fluent aphasia, especially descriptions of Wernicke's aphasic speech and the grammatical structures available to these speakers by taking into account a variety of test results and clinical observations. Test material is used extensively in research and in clinical practice and, as we will see in chapter 2, informs our views of fluent aphasic speech. However, the nature of the speech elicited and the assumptions that arise from assessment depend to a greater or lesser extent on the methods used in testing. Chapter 3 contains a discussion about the nature of testing, a variety of methodologies, and how a theoretical stance influences both methodology and interpretation of results. In chapter 4, I will present a characterisation of the speech of Wernicke's aphasia gathered from analyses of spontaneous speech samples. Some of these are from previously published studies and some are from new clinical studies at the University of Reading. I am indebted to the discussion I have had with colleagues and especially while working with Cindy Thompson and her associates at the Aphasia Research laboratory, Northwestern University, USA, and acknowledge their contribution to my thoughts on analysis.

A brief description is given of agrammatism in chapter 1. In chapter 5, I examine descriptions that claim that agrammatism is a syntactic deficit and distinct from paragrammatism. This is a well-established view in the research literature but does not persist unchallenged. A contrary view is that these two disorders have much in common. In considering this afresh, we will need to have at least a brief overview of comprehension deficits in Wernicke's aphasic speakers. This is the content of chapter 6.

I am writing this monograph from two viewpoints, the clinical linguist's and the practising clinician's. Although the main aim of this book is to provide a new and more detailed description of fluent aphasia and, in constructing that description, to explore the nature of the lexical and grammatical deficits, I am always aware of issues of rehabilitation. Some readers may wonder how these deficits impact upon patients' lives. My experience is that those working in aphasiology but not engaged with aphasia therapy are interested in how aphasia affects the person as a whole. While these matters are not the focus of this monograph, our understanding of fluent aphasia can be enhanced by considering issues that go beyond data and theory. In chapter 7, I describe one speaker with fluent aphasia and his test results, and touch briefly on how these motivated therapy. These data allow us to consider language change in this type of aphasia and how one aphasic speaker coped with his reduced communicative capacities. In chapter 8, I endeavour to bring all these themes together presenting a description of the speech of those with Wernicke's aphasia.

1 *Fluent aphasia: identification and classic descriptions*

Uh we're in the in the kermp kerken kitchen in in the kitchen and there's a lady doing the slowing. She's got the pouring the plate watching it with with um. The water is balancing in the sink the (X) of the sink and the water is pouring all over the bowing bowing all over it.

Introduction

The text quoted above is a small section of a person's description of a picture of a woman washing dishes. The speaker has fluent aphasia. Fluent aphasia is an acquired language disorder that arises subsequent to brain damage. This chapter provides an introduction to the condition and a historical perspective.

Fluent aphasia is a distressing condition for the person who has it and for relatives and friends of that person. It is a relatively common type of aphasia, although there is little published about it compared with the literature on Broca's aphasia. Kertesz (1982:7) described Wernicke's aphasia as 'a common aphasic impairment' and Wallesch, Bak and Schulle-Mouting (1992) found that the majority of patients who survived for one year post-trauma had fluent aphasia. It is also one of the most common types of aphasia found in the first few weeks post trauma (Blanken, Dittmann, Grimm, Marshall and Wallesch 1993). Approximately a quarter of all referrals to our local hospital clinics are diagnosed as fluent aphasia by the speech and language therapist, but at our clinic at the University of Reading, approximately 80 per cent of all adult clients referred with aphasia have fluent aphasia.

Typically, this distressing condition presents problems for the hospital-based rehabilitation team because, for the majority of those referred, their problems are not physical but linguistic. Referrals to our university clinic often arise because it is not at all clear how rehabilitation or support is best provided. Fortunately, people with fluent aphasia are usually mobile in that they can get in and out of cars or on and off buses and therefore can make the journey to a university clinic without specialised transport. For some, though, the severity

5

of the language deficit makes independent travel impossible and they need to travel with a companion. Others, who are less impaired, may also always have a travelling companion, as spouses or carers may be reluctant to see them travel alone because of the language difficulty. Nevertheless, some complete journeys successfully and this is important in terms of rehabilitation and adds to a sense of independence. In some ways, then, people with fluent aphasia make an ideal group to refer on to a clinic situated on a large university campus. My knowledge of normal and aphasic language has been enhanced by working with this group of patients at our University clinic as well as within acute and rehabilitation services.

The identification and description of fluent aphasia occurred relatively late. Although descriptions of aphasia have been around for a very long time, at least since 400 BC, records of the disorder have concentrated on the type of aphasia in which production of words and sentences is seriously disturbed but comprehension remains intact, what is now known as Broca's aphasia. There seem to be no descriptions that match what is now recognised as fluent aphasia (Benton and Joynt 1960). It was not until the nineteenth century and the work of Carl Wernicke, a German neuro-psychiatrist, that a language disorder in which speech production was fluent, although often meaningless, was described. Fluent aphasia is the term I have chosen to use for this type of aphasia, a type that is recognised clinically, although difficult to delineate with a set of agreed criteria. The term 'fluent' refers to the characteristic noted by Wernicke and taken by Goodglass (one of the outstanding aphasiologists of the twentieth century) to be *the* defining characteristic of a group of aphasias. The speech of fluent aphasia is at a normal rate without the effort and hesitation associated with non-fluent aphasia. It is, however, often meaningless.

Taxonomy

Fluent aphasia needs to be thought about within the context of other aphasias, which I will now briefly summarise. (Those readers who are familiar with the field might wish to omit the next couple of paragraphs. For more detailed accounts of different aphasia types, the reader is referred to Goodglass 1993.) There are various ways of grouping aphasia types. This brief résumé is based on what is known as the 'neoclassical' school. This taxonomy has been used by a group of researchers publishing in the latter half of the twentieth century and it is 'neoclassical' in that it is based and refers back to terms used by nineteenth-century aphasiologists. The term 'fluent' denoted an important subdivision of the aphasias and is used in the neoclassical terminology. The fluent/non-fluent division is especially associated with the 'Boston School', a group of clinicians and researchers, led by Harold Goodglass, at the Veterans' Hospital in Boston, USA. In the middle of the twentieth century, Goodglass and colleagues (Goodglass, Quadfasel and Timberlake 1964, Howes and Gerschwind 1964) observed that a major division between two types of aphasia could be made by a simple metric, namely, 'phrase length'. This became the basic feature by which two major groups of aphasias were distinguished. Each of these groups was then further subdivided.

Four types of aphasia are considered to be 'fluent' in the neoclassical classification scheme. These are *Wernicke's aphasia, conduction aphasia, transcortical sensory aphasia and anomia*, of which Wernicke's and conduction aphasia are the most common. Speech in transcortical sensory aphasia and conduction aphasia is fluent, as is the speech in Wernicke's aphasia. Characteristically, patients with conduction aphasia are differentiated from other types of fluent aphasia by their poor repetition abilities, while speakers with transcortical sensory aphasia are good at repeating speech. Comprehension is compromised in conduction aphasia and in transcortical sensory aphasia but less severely than in Wernicke's aphasia. (Classically, comprehension in conduction aphasia has been assumed to be intact although a number of studies from the latter half of the last century have demonstrated that this is not the case.) In conduction aphasia, the comprehension deficit is not as extreme as in Wernicke's aphasia and there are typically more errors in word form. Paraphasic errors, where phoneme substitutions occur, are commonly associated with this disorder. Conduction aphasia occurs rarely (de Bleser 1988:166). Although there is some agreement that lesions that result in Wernicke's aphasia involve the posterior perisylvian speech area, a variety of lesion sites have been reported for all aphasia types (Rapcsak and Rubens 1994). A type of fluent aphasia, often similar to transcortical sensory aphasia, can be observed in senile dementia, further undermining the notion of an isomorphic relationship between lesion site and language disorder. It would appear that there are a number of similarities, such as confusion with word selection and problems following commands, but the overall clinical picture differs. We discuss this further below.

All aphasic speakers (those with fluent and non-fluent aphasia) have difficulties with accessing lexical items. The diagnosis of anomia is given when this feature is predominant, and when comprehension is good or near normal and delivery of speech is fluent. These aphasic speakers have special difficulty in accessing nouns whereas they have less difficulty in accessing verbs. Patients who make a good recovery from either a fluent or non-fluent aphasia may have a persisting residual anomia.

Two or three types of non-fluent aphasia are recognised. The most widely discussed and researched is Broca's aphasia. This is generally associated with lesions in the pre-Rolandic area of the left cerebral cortex. Speech production is reduced and grammar and access to vocabulary is compromised but comprehension is mainly intact. Speech typically consists of short utterances in which grammatical features such as determiners, auxiliary verbs and verb inflections are not always present in obligatory positions. Agrammatism is a term applied by some researchers to Broca's aphasia. For others, agrammatism constitutes a subgroup of Broca's patients who, as well as having production deficits, have problems understanding sentences with certain syntactic structures, specifically when sentence constituents have been moved from their canonical position. Strong claims have been made about the nature of these comprehension deficits (Grodzinsky 1990, 1995, 2000a and b): this condition is explored further in chapter 5.

A much less common non-fluent aphasia is transcortical motor aphasia. People with this type of aphasia have impoverished output, poor ability to produce either single words (in a naming task) or sentences. But, like their sensory counterparts, they are good at repeating both single words and sentences although Rapcsak and Rubens (1994:301) claim that this ability does not extend to repeating sentences with complex grammatical structures. Some researchers (e.g. de Bleser 1988 and Goodglass and Kaplan 1983) include global aphasia in the non-fluent category. People with global aphasia have severe impairment of both production and comprehension. Whether a lack of speech can be considered to be non-fluent is questionable but need not trouble us here. These then are the traditional categories or syndromes. Although they 'leak' in that characteristics are not exclusive to each syndrome, the concept of syndrome serves as a useful shorthand for constellations of features. I will be referring to these syndromes from now on and will use one further distinguishing feature, *fluency versus non-fluency*.

The use of *fluency/non-fluency* as a diagnostic criterion is not universally accepted. Poeck (1989) claimed that the dichotomy created merely reflects the idea that there are basically two distinct types of aphasia, *expressive* and *receptive*, *motor* and *sensory*, or, *Broca's* and *Wernicke's*. This idea, he says, has been around since Wernicke's early publications alerted the field to a type of aphasia which contrasted with Broca's. Despite criticisms, I find the concept of fluent versus non-fluent to have both clinical and pedagogic merit and it will serve as a good starting point. It is a metric that not only divides the aphasic population into two categories which fit, by and large, clinical observations of surface features, but also relates to the neuro-anatomical claims about aphasia advanced by the two nineteenth-century giants of aphasia, Paul Broca and Carl Wernicke. However, this descriptor does not take us very far along the route of considering the linguistic and especially the grammatical features of aphasia. In order to gain some historical perspective, I will start at the beginning, with Wernicke's description of the condition.

Wernicke's aphasia

In 1874 a German neurologist, Carl Wernicke, published a monograph *Aphasia Symptom Complex* in which he described a language disorder found subsequent to brain damage. This language disorder was strikingly different from the aphasia that Paul Broca had described ten years earlier. The aphasic speakers described by Wernicke had copious fluent speech, unlike the slow, halting, non-fluent and sparse aphasic speech described by Broca. Despite the fluency of speech observed by Wernicke, there were obvious problems with word retrieval and, as a consequence, meaning was diminished to a greater or lesser degree. The second distinguishing feature of these speakers was their conspicuous problem with understanding language despite their having normal hearing. Although the presence of deficient understanding was new and perhaps the most remarkable of his observations at the time, Wernicke also noted that impairments of speech were different from those observed by Broca.

Wernicke's 1874 monograph differed from the usual format in that his clinical findings were used to support his attempts to construct a model to explain the processes involved in aphasia (Eggert 1977:21). Wernicke was interested in the representation of language, the storage of images, the creation of lexical memory and the relationship between mental processes and neural structures. Although Wernicke's primary interest in this condition centred on the relationship between mental imagery, memory and the representation and retrieval of words, and it is in this domain that his discussion is focused, there was recognition that the structure of language was disrupted. Wernicke referred to this type of aphasia as *sensory aphasia*. There have been numerous classification schemes proposed and various labels suggested since that time but the term that predominates is, not surprisingly, Wernicke's aphasia.

Wernicke identified two further types of aphasia that arose subsequent to cortical damage in the post-Sylvian area of the brain: transcortical sensory aphasia and conduction aphasia, both of which were similarly characterised by fluent speech. All three types of aphasia are recognised today and (with some minor variations) the same terminology is used both clinically and in much of the research literature. Our understanding of these three types of fluent aphasia has progressed in fits and starts in the intervening years but, as we shall see below, the descriptions used today bear an uncanny resemblance to the descriptions offered by Wernicke.

Wernicke's descriptions arose from his observations of a series of patients who had language disturbances following cortical damage with various aetiologies. Site of lesion was verified post-mortem. He brought attention to language disturbances that resulted from damage to the post-Rolandic cortex. In his 1874 monograph, Wernicke observed that aphasia in some patients resulted in impaired auditory comprehension despite the preserved ability of auditory perception. What was striking was that this deficit was associated with lesions in the left temporal lobe, as was the condition described by Broca. But, importantly, these two types of aphasia were distinguished, from the beginning, by the presence or absence of comprehension deficit and the two contrasting types of abnormal speech.

Wernicke did not actually list the characteristics of the aphasia he was observing but, in a review of Wernicke's work, Eggert (1977:47) notes that the symptom triad that characterises Wernicke's aphasia includes auditory comprehension loss, paraphasia and word-finding impairments. *Paraphasia* is a term that is frequently used in connection with Wernicke's aphasia but seldom defined satisfactorily. Word-finding difficulties are widely recognised as features of all types of fluent aphasia, although here Eggert notes that they are the 'chief characteristic of the final stages of sensory aphasia' (p. 54). 'Final stage' might refer to the mildest type of fluent aphasia or a late stage of recovery: the meaning is not clear. The presence of word-finding difficulties does not separate this type of aphasia from Broca's aphasia or, for that matter, any other type of aphasia. All aphasic speakers have difficulties with word retrieval. The class of word affected may be a distinguishing feature although the distinction probably a lot less categorical than has been suggested in the past (Luzzatti, Raggi, Zonca, Pistarini, Contardi and Pinna 2002).

Wernicke noted two essential features of what he called sensory aphasia. First, there was a loss of word sound perception and hence of access to word meaning. He observed that this loss of understanding was not caused by deafness, for these patients couldn't access meaning through other modalities. The second important symptom of this group of patients was that 'articulate speech remained intact' and, unlike the aphasia described by Broca a few years before, these speakers were 'surprisingly verbose' (Wernicke 1906:226–7, cited in Eggert 1977). Wernicke described these patients as having 'a fairly extensive fund of words' and 'appropriate sentence constructions'. However, speech was impaired. He said that they made 'errors in the choice of expression' and that 'incorrect or transposed words (were) . . . frequent'. He recognised that in severe cases 'distortion of words in speech may degenerate into unintelligibility' commonly known, Wernicke observed, as jargon aphasia (p. 226–7). (All quotes and page numbers relating to Wernicke's work are taken from the translation by Eggert 1977.)

The clinical descriptions given by Wernicke are a key in understanding why the descriptive label of 'fluent' has proved to be so useful despite the lack of a satisfactory definition. Patients with this type of aphasia sound very different from those with Broca's aphasia. There is considerable variation within the clinical population and considerable doubt about boundaries, yet archetypal fluent aphasic speakers are easy to identify despite variations between patients. The variation in the types of symptoms exhibited and the severity of these symptoms has been recognised since the first description offered by Wernicke. In his 1874 monograph he states 'the great variability of the clinical picture of aphasia moves between the two extremes of pure motor aphasia and the pure sensory form' (p. 119).

Furthermore he states that 'although pure motor aphasia has been so thoroughly reviewed in the literature that its relation to involvement of the first frontal convolution is no longer questioned, the pure sensory form on the contrary, to my knowledge has not been represented by a single typical case in the literature' (p. 119). In this monograph, Wernicke described ten cases, the first two of which he considered presented the 'characteristics' and 'primary symptoms of sensory aphasia' (p. 124). The first case, which he described in more detail than the second, is probably nearest to what we would recognise today as typical of Wernicke's aphasia.

> *4) The patient described is a woman of 59 years who suddenly became ill. She was observed to comprehend 'absolutely nothing'; 'her answers to questions were inappropriate'; the sentences were 'incorrectly produced, containing meaningless and garbled words'. Despite this, the meaning of the sentence 'could be grasped in a general way'. Although her inability to answer questions gave the superficial appearance of dementia, her behaviour was 'calm and appropriate'. She had severe dysgraphia and was unable to read. Her comprehension improved rapidly and there was some improvement in her speech although she remained aphasic.*

Here the essential elements of sensory aphasia are exhibited: diminished comprehension, impaired language production, agraphia and alexia, although we are not told whether the patient was literate prior to her illness. Wernicke notes that 'superficially she gave the impression of dementia' (p. 120). Although there are some patients with fluent aphasia who, even today, are misdiagnosed as demented rather than aphasic, it is difficult to gauge what Wernicke was commenting on. It may have been the speaker's disordered language, for he also observed that her behaviour was 'calm and appropriate'.

Today, a clear clinical distinction is made between patients who have fluent aphasia and may seem confused because they cannot follow instructions, and those who have behavioural as well as language disturbances (for example, patients with multi-infarct dementia). Wernicke did not make this distinction at all clear in his 1874 monograph. Of the ten cases that he describes, at least three suffer from some kind of dementia in addition to their aphasia. One of these cases and two of the others are reported to have died within a short period. So this collection of patients does not represent a collection of patients with the archetypal sensory aphasia he was suggesting existed. Nor did Wernicke intend it to. The subtitle of this monograph is *a psychological study on an anatomical basis* that indicates Wernicke's interest in making connections between deficits and site of lesion and his discipline of psychiatry.

From these first descriptions it has been assumed that while the comprehension impairment is unspecified, the major locus of difficulties in language production is lexical while grammar remains unimpaired. Despite this, grammatical errors have been noted from Wernicke onwards. Kleist (1916, cited by Butterworth, Panzeri, Semenza and Ferren 1990) introduced the notion of paragrammatism which was, and remains, ill-defined, with definitions such as 'confused and incomplete but not necessarily simplified constructions' (Goodglass and Hunt 1958). Butterworth et al. (1990) use the descriptive phrase 'confused and erroneous grammatical structures' in the introduction to their study. Following the analyses used by Butterworth and Howard (1987) for four English aphasic speakers, they provide a detailed description of one Italian speaker with paragrammatism. Both accounts detail a number of errors with closed-class and open-class words and problems with sentence construction.

An example of fluent aphasia

We will now look at some aphasic data taken from samples collected from a patient who has attended the speech and language therapy clinic at the University of Reading for a number of years. It will provide data that can be compared with the examples given by Wernicke. We will return to consider this speaker's language deficits in much more detail in later chapters.

The subject

The subject, MG, was 54 when he had a sudden stroke and became aphasic. He has no obvious physical disabilities, he talks fluently, at a normal rate using normal intonation patterns. He responds to the normal conventions of social interaction such as attempting greetings and inquiring after the welfare of others. During these exchanges he makes good use of social phrases and it takes a few moments after first meeting him to realise that he is aphasic. His language deficits become apparent when he talks at length or is asked questions. The following is part of his description of what happened in the first few months following the stroke. It reveals some of the difficulties he has:

> (1) *I went home from the Bath Hospital* [he gives the incorrect name of the hospital] *and I couldn't at all . . . no . . nothing at all . . . no . . . absolutely nothing . . . I went down to the HXX* [gives the name of his consultant] *you know* [therapist checks name of consultant neurologist] *Mr HXXX yes . . . yes and he (er) he he said to me well . . . I look . . . I went home from the Bath Hospital* [he gives the incorrect name of the hospital] *. . . and I couldn't at all no . . nothing at all no . . . absolutely nothing . . . I went down to the HXX* [gives the correct name of his consultant neurologist again] *you know . . . and he said he said (er) I think I'll do you he said . . . can you . . . can you do something about it I said . . . nothing he said (er) . . . I'll just say have have you any cakes today that's what he said . . . have you any cakes today . . . yeah . . . that's what he said . . . and blank . . . I couldn't do it at all . . . nothing . . . absolutely nothing . . .* [therapist asks when the incident happened] *. . . seven years ago . . . and so I went back to the X Hospital* [gives correct name of a different hospital] *and it's a long hard job I can tell you*

This conversation took place seven years after the onset of aphasia and after some recovery had occurred. Nevertheless, although the rate of delivery and the intonation used sounds normal, the speaker's ability to communicate remains impaired, as revealed above, and his language remains typical of fluent aphasia. For example, the reported exchange between him and the consultant:

> (2)   *'I think I'll do you he said can you can you do something about it I said'*

Although comprising two well-formed sentences (ignoring the repetition), the utterance is meaningless as the utterance lacks referents. One might guess what MG was trying to say but there is nothing in the surrounding utterances that would confirm speculations. As it stands, *I think I'll do you* not only makes no sense but is highly implausible. He recognises the demands of the discourse and tries to answer the therapist's questions but his response is more or less meaningless. The therapist's limited understanding of this exchange depended on her knowledge of background information, the topic, the names of the hospital, the consultant and some details of MG's past history. If his conversational partner had not had this information the exchange would have been considerably less successful.

Applying Wernicke's description to candidate cases

Applying Wernicke's observations to this sample, we see that the speech is clear in that there are no sound distortions or substitutions. This supports Wernicke's observation that 'articulate speech' is intact. While MG is able to form simple sentences (*so I went back to the hospital*), there are no examples of embedding in this sample and he backtracks and repeats himself. He uses a range of words, the major lexical categories, nouns, verbs, and adjectives, as well as determiners, prepositions and auxiliary verbs. Whether Wernicke would judge MG as having 'appropriate' sentences and an 'extensive fund of words' is uncertain as no criteria are given for 'appropriate' or for 'extensive'. The same problem arises if the characteristic of verbosity, a notoriously subjective quality, is considered. Taking just these descriptors, 'articulate speech', 'appropriate sentences', 'extensive fund of words' and 'verbosity', MG matches Wernicke's description of sensory aphasia.

In terms of deficits, it can be seen without further analyses that there are problems with lexical access resulting in omissions and substitutions. These involve proper nouns, (the names of the hospital and his consultant), a lexical verb (*I couldn't nothing at all*) and a verb argument (*I look*). There would seem to be a reduction in the range of lexical verbs with *do* used, probably, inappropriately on at least two occasions (*I'll think I'll do you*; *I couldn't do it at all*). There are, possibly, other lexical substitutions that go undetected in spontaneous speech. He uses the determiner *the* before the surname of his consultant. This may be an error of addition or an error of substitution where the surname of the consultant has been substituted for the name of the hospital. There are no apparent errors in inflectional morphology in this example and no other obvious indications that the speaker does not have access to grammar. He is able to use simple declarative sentences, negation (*I couldn't do it at all*), and one question structure (*have you any cakes?*).

There are some similarities between MG's speech and that of a patient, Mrs A, the second patient described by Wernicke. Here is a sample of conversational speech translated by Eggert (1977) as follows:

(3)   DR WERNICKE: *I would like to know how old you are.*
       MRS A.:   *Yes, that I don't know at all. What my name (Wie ich so
                      hieszen schwiere)* [She has obvious difficulties and
                      attempts to correct herself.] *what I'm called hear/here* [in
                      German *hore*]
       DR WERNICKE: *Would you perhaps give me your hand?*
       MRS A.:   *I don't know how I* [Presents no trace of comprehension]
       DR WERNICKE: *Where is Richard?*
       MRS A.:   [she thinks for a long time] *My sodom (neologism) my
                      Richard*
       DR WERNICKE: *Do you need anything?*
       MRS A.:   *Oh my, now who would anyone say something to me*

If this is a true account of a conversation between a consultant and his confused and recently aphasic patient, then it is a very strange one. From the script given, it would seem that Wernicke jumped from topic to topic giving the patient very little time to work out what was required of her. The patient seems to be confused by the questioning and this confusion is compounding her production errors. Even so, we can see that, like MG, she has difficulties with lexical access (*sodom* for 'son') and even if she doesn't have problems formulating sentences, then certainly there are problems with forming meaningful sentences.

No autopsy information is given about this patient although it is Wernicke's second case which Eggert (p. 91) considers (with cases one and eight) 'demonstrate(s) the clinical symptoms of sensory aphasia', the syndrome we now call Wernicke's aphasia. However, although case one could be recognised today as a Wernicke's aphasic, I would consider neither case two nor case eight as good examples of Wernicke's aphasia. Case two was a 75-year-old woman, who appeared demented on admission to hospital. She used 'mutilated' and 'transposed' words and had severe problems in understanding, which could be typical of a Wernicke's aphasia, yet she 'paid little attention to her surroundings, and in keeping with the severity of her illness, showed little desire to converse', which is not typical. She died two months after admission to hospital. Autopsy revealed extensive cerebral damage and 'included the gyri and island regions in both hemispheres'. There was damage to the first temporal gyrus, as Eggert notes (p. 91), but the extent of the damage in other areas of the brain does not permit this case to be seen as a good exemplar of the relationship between temporal lobe damage and Wernicke's aphasia.

The citation of case eight as one who demonstrated the clinical symptoms of sensory aphasia is puzzling. It is true that this patient was also found to have temporal lobe damage but there was other cerebral damage that would be expected given the severity of her symptoms. She had a complete right hemiplegia and some involvement of the facial nerve. Speech was reported to be limited to 'yes' and she was said to understand nothing. Contrary to Eggert's claims, this case would be clinically classified today as a global aphasia, that is a profound aphasia affecting all modalities.

Descriptions in the twentieth century: the Boston School

Probably the most widely used taxonomy, one that is referred to extensively in research and clinical literature, is that developed by Goodglass and his colleagues (Goodglass and Kaplan 1972, 1983, Goodglass, Kaplan and Baresi 2001). A number of taxonomies were developed during the second half of the last century (Kertesz 1982) but the terms used for the major aphasia categories and the descriptions given have remained fairly constant. There have, not surprisingly, been some changes in the explanations offered as more has been learnt about language and language processes. Goodglass (whom Marshall (1995:307) described as 'the grand old man of aphasiology'), claims that the modern taxonomy of aphasia contains 'a major polarity in symptomatology' between 'those patients who are unable to string words into grammatically organised phrases or sentences and those who cannot supply the information-carrying nouns and verbs' (1993:6). The former group, the agrammatic, is further characterised by Goodglass as 'lacking in small grammatical words such as prepositions, auxiliary verbs and articles'. The latter type of aphasia he identifies as anomia. The distinction here seems to be one of lexical access rather than grammatical ability, for, despite the claim that agrammatic patients cannot form sentences, he goes on to state that they 'typically use one-to-three-word noun phrases or verb phrases to express themselves'.

Leaving aside for the moment the confusion about the type of phrases identified here, the focus would seem to be on the differential retrieval of items from the lexicon rather than the computational aspect of language. The inability to 'string words into grammatically organised phrases or sentences' equates with a problem with grammar while those who 'cannot supply the information-carrying nouns and verbs' is found in those who have an intact grammar. At this stage, there is no mention of Wernicke's or conduction aphasia, two forms of fluent aphasia, but the diagnostic features now seem to be the presence of lexical and syntactic deficits rather than the fluency dimension which was used in Goodglass' earlier taxonomies.

This 'major polarity' is not based on intact versus damaged grammars. Indeed, Goodglass (1993:102) argues against 'syntax as an undifferentiated psychological capacity that can be damaged or spared as a unit'. This is pretty uncontroversial but, nevertheless, crucial for syndromic position where syndromes are recognised by different patterns of deficit. Goodglass concentrates on describing surface manifestations of agrammatic aphasia, which he typifies as having short sentences and loss of inflectional morphology. Non-fluency, once a defining feature, is now said to be common but not an essential feature. Deficits of various aspects of the grammar, as he sees it, are now the essential defining features (p. 106). This is somewhat at variance with the earlier statements about the lexical retrieval deficits but we will move on to his characterisation of fluent aphasia and the feature of paragrammatism.

Here, again, while discussing the dimension of fluency, Goodglass concentrates on the 'impression on the listener' and describes the speech as 'normal or hyper-fluent, with natural speech prosody' (p. 108). As far as the grammar is concerned, he notes that there is 'no lack of morphology'. A variety of sentence structures are found in fluent aphasia. Although there is a tendency for sentence structures to be 'reduced on average', embedding does occur. Although impairment of lexical accessing affects the open rather than the closed class words, omissions and substitutions of grammatical morphemes also occur. Goodglass considers that both agrammatism and paragrammatism 'affect the same language domain' (p. 108) and that paragrammatism may involve 'incoherent and aimless' syntactic structures with 'nouns appearing in verb slots' and vice versa. Thus it would appear that he considers grammatical deficits can occur in both non-fluent and fluent aphasia, but there will be different types of deficit in the different types of syndromes.

This is an important distinction and at odds with the notion that non-fluent and fluent aphasia are impairments to separate domains of language. If grammar is compromised in both paragrammatic and agrammatic language, as these terms would imply, then the idea that domains of language have distinct cortical representation is compromised for each domain of language. Grammar on the one hand and lexis on the other are, broadly speaking, associated with anterior and posterior lesions respectively. But if grammatical deficits occur in both types of aphasia, grammar cannot be represented only within a circumscribed area of the frontal lobe. We discuss this issue in greater detail below.

The Boston School has been a strong advocate of localisation, but here Goodglass seems to be emphasising that, for diagnostic purposes, that is, deciding which type of aphasia is present, the prime consideration is performance, namely how the person speaks and what level of comprehension is present. This approach has clinical validity. There is a clear distinction to be made between the speech in Wernicke's and Broca's aphasia. However, a number of questions remain: what is the nature of the deficit in each syndrome; what is the underlying nature; what are the defining characteristics; how distinct are the syndromes? These questions remain over twenty years since the classification system was developed. The descriptions offered barely touch on these points but, as they offer good operational definitions of different types of aphasia, they remain important.

Goodglass and Wernicke's aphasia

Goodglass provides a description of Wernicke's aphasia: 'speech output is facile in articulation and sentence structure, tending to be filled with ill-chosen words and poorly formed sentences', 'word finding is severely restricted so that free conversation is often circumlocutory and empty', 'rate of speech is sometimes excessively rapid' (p. 210). Here again, the essential features are:

> 1) a normal (or excessive) rate of speech; 2) problems of lexical access especially for open class words which is manifested by selection errors of various types; 3) errors in inflectional morphology; 4) use of well-formed sentences although there may be some problems with sentence formulation and reduction in sentence complexity.

Wernicke's aphasic speakers are also identified by their defective comprehension of spoken and written language. They are considered to be generally unaware of their production errors.

Other twentieth-century descriptions of fluent aphasia

Damasio (1981:56) regarded fluency as a 'helpful category' and, while observing that the term could mean 'different things to different authors', proposed that fluency was generally taken to convey that the non-segmental features of rate and intonation were normal. Yet as for calibrating this feature, he suggested that it could be measured not by rate or intonation but by 'the longest string of words'. Kertesz (1982) describes Wernicke's aphasia as 'copious, fluent, prosodically correct (language), resembling English syntax and inflection'. He also put considerable emphasis on fluency, considering it to be an important diagnostic feature. Like Goodglass and Kaplan, he developed a scoring system whereby the clinician could arrive at a fluency rating. However, the ten-point scale has such a hotchpotch of items that any notion of 'fluency' referring to something like a collection of super-segmental features flies out of the window. For example, it includes scoring for the presence or absence of 'recurrent utterances', 'stereotypic utterances', 'mumbling, very low jargon', 'circumlocution', 'mostly complete sentences' and finally, to achieve maximal scores 'sentences of normal length and complexity, without any perceptible word-finding difficulty' (p. 41). So what might have been developed as a useful metric with, for example, well-defined categories of intonation patterns and rate of speech, was, instead, taken up as a very general all-purpose measure of 'normal' production. Such metrics that bundled together aspects of language that can be differentially impaired did nothing to assist in clinical diagnosis. Enterprises which set out to try and clarify the diagnostic confusion in fact added to it.

Harley (1995:270) describes Wernicke's aphasic speech as 'fluent but often meaningless . . . speech forms (sic) well-formed sentences with copious grammatical elements and with normal prosody . . . there are obvious major content word-finding difficulties'. He supports the classical view of a dissociation between 'syntactic planning and grammatical element retrieval' (typical of Broca's aphasia) and 'content word retrieval' (impaired in Wernicke's type but intact in Broca's type). For Harley, the deficits displayed in Wernicke's aphasia can be interpreted as problems with the semantic-phonological access system, but whether he envisages retrieval difficulties to be both semantic and phonological or whether he interprets lexical errors as either semantic or phonological is not clear. He discusses the use of the Garrett's (1975, 1976) model of language production in various accounts of aphasia. (For a more recent account see Garrett 1988.) For example, a study by Schwartz (1987) is given as an example of agrammatism using this model, and Buckingham (1986) is quoted for accounts of lexical errors found in fluent aphasia and especially neologisms. Following the Garrett model of language production, in which distinct non-interactive stages of processing exist, Harley assumes that the greater difficulty with content compared with function words can be explained by the notion that these different types of words are computed at different stages of building a sentence. He claims that function words and grammatical morphemes are added at the Positional level, which is distinct, and perhaps at a later stage than the Functional level, where content words are specified. Harley assumes that 'content words are retrieved independently from their syntactic frames and inflections, and jargon (found in fluent aphasia) is a disorder of lexical retrieval'. Although these stages are probably happening at the same time, the stages are not interactive and thus discrete deficits can be observed. The dissociation between the assumed syntactic deficit of Broca's aphasia and the lexical deficit of Wernicke's aphasia adds, in Harley's view, good support for the model.

There is a tendency for there to be more difficulty with content words, rather than function words, but this difference is not absolute. Thus the distinction is not lexical versus syntactic per se, for the lexical retrieval is also subject to grammatical influence. This undermines Harley's claim that the differences found between Broca's and Wernicke's aphasia supports the dissociation between the production of syntax and the retrieval of lexical forms. In effect, Harley summarises the accepted view that Broca's and Wernicke's aphasia arise following damage to one or other of these two domains of language. He presents his summary in a slightly different way from the Boston School yet maintains this widely accepted distinction. The main deficit of Wernicke's aphasia is, he claims, one of lexical retrieval.

Speakers with fluent aphasia, however, have errors of sentence structure. Davis (2000:117), wisely, hedges his bets. He observes, on the one hand, that 'syntactic aspects of language formulation are *relatively* spared . . . and, thus, are dissociated from lexical aspects' (my italics), while noting, on the other, that paragrammatism, a classical component of Wernicke's aphasia, includes substitution of grammatical morphemes, a feature seemingly ignored by Harley. Furthermore, speakers with Wernicke's aphasia do make the same types of errors as those with Broca's aphasia and tend to use less complex sentence structures (Davis 2000). These facts weaken the view that in Broca's and Wernicke's aphasia we see a clear dissociation between syntactic abilities and lexical access. At best, what is seen is a *relative* preservation of one or other of these two components of language, but there is rarely a clear line to be drawn between these two types of aphasia, as the older textbooks like to suggest. Descriptions are now often more cautious. Obler and Gjerlow (1999) observe that the linguistic deficits observed in Wernicke's aphasics *tend* to be more lexical-semantic than those found in Broca's aphasia.

More sophistication?

So how have the descriptions developed in the past thirty years or so? With some notable exceptions, descriptions of Wernicke's aphasia agree on the perceived fluency. They acknowledge that lexical retrieval problems exist and seriously compromise the ability to convey meaning and that sentence formulation may be disrupted, but there has been little advance in providing a more detailed and systematic description. Terms used in descriptions are still not defined and may be used in a seemingly contradictory fashion. Goodglass, describing Wernicke's speech, states that '[they] can string words and phrases into organised phrases and sentences' yet they have 'poorly formed sentences', that there is 'no lack of morphemes' but then there is 'omission and substitution of grammatical morphemes'. What does this mean? Here, 'morphemes' may refer to lexical or grammatical morphemes and, within the category of grammatical morphemes, bound or free forms. If it refers to bound forms, then a distinction can be drawn between inflectional morphemes such as those used to signal tense and agreement, (*jump, jumps, jumped*) and derivational morphemes (*beauty/beautiful*). Speakers with Wernicke's aphasia do make errors with both lexical morphemes (lexical semantic errors) and grammatical morphemes (inflectional errors) although errors in grammatical morphemes occur less frequently than they do in non-fluent aphasia. The picture is complicated by other descriptions. Benson and Ardila (1996) describe Wernicke's aphasic speech as 'fluent with normal or excessive number of words produced (logorrhea) produced with normal articulation and prosody. The grammatical structure of the verbal output is adequate but it can contain an excess of grammatical morphemes (paragrammatism)' (p. 144). It is puzzling to imagine what an 'excessive' number of grammatical morphemes might sound like.

There is a suggestion that frequently occurs in the literature that somehow patients with Wernicke's aphasia talk too much, have 'logorrhea' or are 'hyper-fluent' or 'verbose'. Speakers with Wernicke's aphasia may not be as good at taking conversational turns as normal speakers, may hold the floor longer and be poor at self-monitoring. There is little evidence, however, that rate of speech is excessive. (This will be further discussed in chapter 2). The notion of too many grammatical morphemes is also somewhat bizarre. Presumably, what the observers are commenting on is the disproportionate number of closed-class words compared with open-class words, but no supporting evidence is given. Later in this monograph we will examine this claim using analyses of continuous fluent aphasia speech. What we will observe is not so much a change in proportion of word types but a change in proportion of correctly selected word types. We shall note the absence of the use of multiple grammatical morphemes attached to the same stem, an error that never, in my experience, occurs.

Syndromes

We have touched upon the unsatisfactory nature of descriptions of Wernicke's aphasia and have been alerted to the variation found in this syndrome. One reason for this dissatisfaction could be that the clinical concept of syndrome does not match psychological reality and that there is too much variation in the language deficits for patients to be divided into types or syndromes. A syndrome is considered to be a condition that (a) has an identifiable cluster of features that co-occur and that (b) these features arise from the same cause. So, for example, Down's syndrome is recognised by clinical features (e.g. certain physical characteristics), behavioural characteristics (slow maturation, learning difficulties), which, for this syndrome, all arise as a consequence of a genetic abnormality (abnormalities in chromosome 21). All people identified with Down's syndrome will have all these features, although with varying degrees of severity. Aphasiologists, following a medical model, have endeavoured to divide the range of language deficits observed in aphasia into entities and label these 'syndromes'. This approach, based on the work of the nineteenth-century neurologists, persists and the influence is strong, especially in the United States of America and in much of the empirical research focused on defining the nature of the language deficit in aphasia.

In clinical practice it is common to find that a large number of patients do not fit into any of the neoclassical syndromes, and syndrome diagnosis does not play a major part in many clinical assessments. In fact, Albert, Goodglass, Helm, Rubens and Alexander (1981), agreeing with the findings of Prins, Snow and Wagenaar (1978) state that only 20–30 per cent of patients can be satisfactorily allocated to a syndrome. Kertesz (1982), using a modified scheme, found that only a small proportion fitted his syndromes. These findings are clearly a major problem for those advocating the continuous use of the Boston taxonomy. Yet classifying by syndrome persists and, despite the widespread dissatisfaction with a syndromic classification scheme, the quest to provide a test format which will lead to a diagnosis continues unabated with an English adaptation of the Aachen Aphasia Test, a test designed to allocate patients to defined subgroups, currently under way (Huber, Poeck and Willmes 1984:291; Miller, Willmes and de Bleser 2000). Test development tends to divide into those tests that strive to perfect a mode of classifying patients, as in the Aachen, and those that focus on an in-depth analysis of one or two aspects of aphasia. The former are likely to continue to be used for large numbers of patients and research subjects in order to establish a common currency while the specialised probe instruments allow the clinician or experimenter to explore the nature of aphasia with individuals or small groups. Individual 'bespoke' tailoring of patient profiles is great but, for many, off-the-shelf diagnosis is not only utilitarian but also helps to put each new patient or research subject into a broad category.

It is generally true that those developing such classifications and diagnostic tests look at surface features of language, especially at errors, and the association between the surface features and the frequency of errors. The purpose had not been to relate the aphasic features to any linguistic or psychological model. In the last twenty years or so, however, there have been big changes of emphasis with researchers working with either psychological or linguistic models seeking to uncover patterns of aphasic errors and to fit these patterns to a theoretical model. Those working with models taken from cognitive psychology have looked at error patterns of individual patients and talked about 'processes' and 'modules'. By and large, the models applied to aphasia have been concerned with single-word processing and the assumed separation of the stages of semantic and phonological form. Applications of such models to aphasia have encouraged single-case studies and an evangelical campaign against the so-called syndromic approach to aphasia and the associated use of group studies.

The alternative camp has argued vigorously in favour of group studies and the entity of well-defined syndromes, the putative example being agrammatism. Within this tradition, various researchers (e.g. Zurif, Swinney, Shapiro, Grodzinsky and their colleagues) have mounted a staunch reply to those who attack the notion of agrammatism as a 'functional entity'. For example, Grodzinsky (1991:556) describes agrammatism as the 'flagship of neuropsychology'. The recognition of this type of aphasia is based on considerable empirical evidence and supported by well-argued theoretical explanations for the pattern of deficits found. Furthermore, there is an assumption that the recognised pattern of deficits arises from damage to a fairly well-circumscribed cortical area, Broca's area, long associated with grammar or at least the computation aspect of language. However, as we will consider below, there is considerable evidence that the relationship between site of lesion and resulting aphasic deficits is far from straightforward, and, recently, Grodzinsky has made an attempt to qualify and limit which bits of language are represented within Broca's area. He has claimed that Broca's area is not responsible for grammar per se, for some grammatical processes continue to function after lesions to Broca's area. Only one grammatical process is implicated and that is a grammatical operation known as trace. This bold claim has met with considerable criticism, some of which fundamentally disagrees with the notion that grammar is damaged. Others challenge details of the claim: for example, the responses to a lead paper in *Behavioral and Brain Sciences* (February 2001) and papers in *Brain and Language (Brain and Language 1995)*. We return to some of these issues in chapter 4.

Subject variation

On-line and off-line language studies using groups engage in a certain amount of 'smoothing' of the data, often excluding 'noise' in the data. What researchers look for is a group result: individual differences are lost. This is common in on-line brain studies and, on the whole, accepted as part of the methodology. The same acceptance is not so readily granted to aphasia studies. Notwithstanding the fact that variation in behaviour is commonplace, the existence of variation within the aphasic population remains a problem for some aphasiologists (e.g. Caramazza and Miceli 1991). These researchers prefer to study individual cases, which, in crude methodological terms, is not too dissimilar from the approach of the nineteenth-century aphasiologists. The single-subject design is considered to be essential by some, claiming that the necessary abstraction which group studies entail is reductionist and involves procedures which produce 'quantitative data . . . that bear little relation to actuality' (Marshall 1995:309). In truth, both approaches add to our knowledge of aphasia.

Syndrome-lesion site relationship

Aphasia arises as a consequence of cerebral damage. A person with aphasia is suffering from symptoms resulting from cerebral trauma. Outside war-zones, most traumas are the result of cerebral vascular accidents, haemorrhages, embolisms, infarcts, infection and other cerebral lesions. The three classic aphasia syndromes known as Broca's, Conduction and Wernicke's aphasia are also known as 'peri-Sylvian aphasic syndromes' as the site of lesion is usually, although not exclusively, in this region. Wernicke's aphasia is associated with lesions in the superior temporal regions of the left cerebral hemisphere, the superior and middle temporal gyri. There are frequently extensions to this region involving the supramarginal/angular gyrus and the lateral, temporal/occipital regions (Benson and Adila 1996). There are also reports of Wernicke's aphasia following subcortical damage (Alexander, Naeser and Palumbo 1987).

The evidence that links site of lesion with specific language deficit is hazy, while the evidence for an isomorphic relationship between site of lesion and aphasic syndrome is very hazy. And, despite the quest to establish this relationship, a quest that has lasted in excess of one hundred years, results continue to be contradictory and opinions sharply divided on the nature of the relationship. The development of a range of advanced methods of neurological investigation, which include computorised tomography, magnetic imaging, electrical stimulation and blood-flow studies, has brought greater information but little clarity. Basso, Lecours, Moraschini and Vanier (1985) and de Bleser (1988) demonstrated that there is, at best, a weak association between site of lesion and syndrome. In de Bleser's study, digital-lesion information from computer tomographs of forty-six subjects was studied. The subjects were chosen from a pool of seventy individuals on the basis of whether they were good or poor exemplars of a syndrome. The Aachen Aphasia Test (Huber, Poeck and Willmes 1984) was used for classification. Two of the 'good' Wernicke's subjects had post-Rolandic lesions and two had lesions in the pre-Rolandic area *as well as* post-Rolandic lesions. Of the other Wernicke subjects who were considered to be good exemplars, seven had post-Rolandic lesions and five had pre-Rolandic lesions. Thus, even when subjects are chosen as good exemplars of their syndrome, sites of lesion may differ and de Bleser concludes that the 'standard assumptions of deficit theory, that a simple one-to-one mapping obtains between brain areas and psychological functions will have to be revised' (p. 184). A study by Willmes and Poeck (1993) investigated the relationship between diagnosis on the Aachen Aphasia Test and lesion site using a series of CT scans. Their findings suggest that Wernicke's aphasia is most likely to arise subsequent to damage in the post-Rolandic area: this was true for 90 per cent of all their subjects. However, a lesion in this area will not inevitably lead to Wernicke's aphasia, a finding supported by Benson and Ardila (1996). Only *48 per cent* of Willmes and Poeck's subjects with lesions in Wernicke's area presented with Wernicke's aphasia, and their cohort contained subjects with persisting Wernicke's aphasia although with, apparently, only small anterior lesions.

Willems and Poeck, while claiming that there is a great variety of language impairment irrespective of the size of the lesion (p. 1538), suggest that these results and those from similar studies be interpreted with caution. They note that there are problems with methodology. They note difficulties with the degree of precision obtained in localising lesions, problems with averaging across groups, the fact that the time of examination may well be crucial yet is seldom accounted for and that symptoms, but presumably not lesion sites, can change over time. Recent studies (Hollis 2002, Hollis and Heidler 2002) have confirmed that the time of testing can be crucial, with quite marked neural changes taking place immediately after the onset of aphasia. Finally, there is a problem in accepting the psychological reality of the syndromes. If a syndrome is poorly defined or doesn't actually exist, then it would indeed be surprising if a relationship were to be found between syndrome and lesion site.

The growing dissatisfaction with the concept of 'syndrome' parallels growth in another approach to the study of the brain–language relationship. While studies that have led to the notion of aphasic syndromes have arisen from a lesion-based framework, a new research paradigm using normal subjects has generated a vast array of new data. In these studies, various sophisticated imaging procedures are used to map brain activity. Investigations may involve subjects performing specific language tasks (usually processing) while electrical stimulation is applied to specific cerebral areas. The assumption here is that the current produces a localised lesion, and deficits in performance that occur during these tasks therefore arise as a consequence of lesioning that region of the brain responsible for the part of the language process that is under investigation. Other procedures use imaging techniques to measure cerebral blood flow. Brain activity is taken to be reflected in the increased blood flow that occurs while normal subjects perform various tasks that are presumed to represent components of language processing. If activity occurs in specific cerebral sites and while tasks are performed, then an assumption is made that that particular site is associated with, or responsible for, that activity.

Studies with normal subjects

Studies motivated by different theoretical stances may use similar methodologies. For example, Wise, Chollet, Hadar, Friston, Hoffner and Frackowiak (1991:1804) set up tasks which they claimed 'encompassed some of the basic elements of language processing' as a way of identifying neural networks that participate in the processing of single words. Their starting point was a theoretical model of language processing (Ellis and Young 1988) in which comprehension is broken down into modules of auditory analysis, that is, matching incoming signals within the auditory input lexicon and within the semantic module. The tasks were designed to tap various levels of the process. Normal subjects were required to listen to various word lists. The first list was of non-words, and subjects were just required to listen. In the next two tasks, subjects were required to listen to lists of word pairs and to make simple semantic judgements about the pairs. In the fourth task, subjects were required to listen to nouns and, as each word was presented, asked to think of as many associated verbs as possible. Activity-related changes in regional cerebral blood flow (rCBF) were measured by positron emission tomography (PET). By subtracting the change in activity from a base-line achieved from the change in activity obtained while the subjects listened to nonsense words, assumptions are made about the location of neural activity for the semantic and verb-generation tasks. The results confirmed that 'word comprehension is a function localised to the superior temporal lobes' (p. 1815). The localisation of brain activity when subjects were processing non-words did not differ from when they were processing real words. There was, however, a significant increase in rCBF in Wernicke's area during the verb-generation task, but during this task some activation in the anterior cerebral regions also occurred. The increase of activation of Wernicke's area in the verb task did not, surprisingly, lead the authors to predict that verbs might be vulnerable in this type of aphasia, although, as we will see later, there is accumulating evidence that suggests this might be the case.

Once again, the results are difficult to interpret. Both listening to non-words and making judgements about real words produced activity in the same cerebral areas. Does this mean that there is no designated location for processing real words or could it mean that the activity of listening to words, whether real or nonsense, produces increased blood flow of such a magnitude that it masked other differences? The increase in brain activity in the anterior regions during the verb-generation task could arise from the special status of this word class, or, because it was the only task that required the subjects to generate words, albeit silently. A number of investigators claim that Broca's area is associated or even 'crucial' to sub-vocal rehearsal (Paulesu, Frith and Frackowiak 1993). If this is accepted, then activation of this area during the verb task is unremarkable and might arise because of sub-vocal rehearsal of words rather than because of some special status of verbs.

The above is an example from the many studies published. Exciting as they are, such studies have acknowledged problems of procedure and interpretation. The data analyses in the Wise et al. study involved standardising for each subject's brain size, normalising and averaging across the six subjects. A certain amount of smoothing of the original scans was also performed (p. 1806). Thus, small variations are lost. As with the work on syndrome-lesion site correlates, it is not at all clear that the tasks generating word lists are representative of the basic elements of language processing as claimed by the authors (p. 1804). Reviewing five studies on phonological processing, Poeppel (1996) challenges the claim that tasks used in such studies are necessarily interpretable as adding to our knowledge about how the language systems are neurologically organised. What we might be observing is the neural organisation required by the experimental tasks.

Similar investigative techniques have been used to address very different issues in language research, which, on the face of it, may appear to investigate aspects of language processing directly. Jaeger, Lockwood, Kemmerer, van Valin, Murphy and Khalak (1996) used a PET study to investigate brain activity associated with producing regular verbs and brain activity associated with producing irregular verbs. They claimed that their results made it clear that 'there are major differences in both the location and the amount of brain activation in the regular versus irregular task' (p. 484) and that the study had demonstrated the value of applying neurolinguistic evidence to controversies in linguistics. Others may judge that these studies do not in fact add very much new information. In the Jaeger study, the nature of the contrasting tasks might have contributed to the differences found. The verb types were not presented in mixed lists, for example, and once again it is a matter of debate as to how far these experimental tasks can inform us about processing connected language.

A later study looking at similar phenomena, regular and irregular verbs and nouns, but using event related functional magnetic resonance imaging (fMRI) (Beretta, Campbell, Carr, Huang, Schmitt, Christianson and Cao 2003), claims to support Jaeger et al.'s finding. Beretta et al. found greater activation of irregular forms than for regular and greater lateralisation to the left hemisphere for the regulars; when significant differences were found within major regions, irregulars gained greater activation than regulars. They conclude that their findings support the dual-route account of inflection, that is, grammatical operations for the regular and lexical memory for the irregular forms.

Poeppel (1996) reviews five studies of phonological processing. All these studies used positron emission tomography to monitor changes in regional cerebral blood flow (rCBF). Poeppel focuses his critique on the rhyme judgement tasks deployed by the researchers to investigate phonological processing. (These were not the only experimental tasks used, as the authors point out in their replies to Poeppel.) Poeppel claims that these studies fail to show that there is either a single area implicated in 'phonetic/phonological processing' or that the areas implicated overlap (p. 321). A trenchant response follows in which the authors of the papers reviewed defend their results by claiming that different areas are activated because of the different nature of the tasks (p. 354) and the different processes the tasks involve (p. 355). They claim that there is an 'impressive amount of convergence of activation found in the left inferior frontal gyrus (p. 357) and, rather differently, that different lesion sites of activation are not unexpected if language functions are 'a vast continuous domain spreading over the left hemispheric peri-Sylvian cortex' (Demonet, Fiez, Paulesu, Petersen and Zatorre 1996:361).

Demonet et al. (1996) quote work on transcortical sensory aphasia by Alexander, Naeser and Palumbo (1989) to support this notion. Alexander and colleagues claim that certain aphasic deficits, in this case lexical semantic comprehension deficits, can arise from different lesions sites because these sites are interconnected into a network which subserves the language functions. They therefore suggest that, because different sites have been implicated in the phonological studies reviewed by Poeppel, this may point away from the notion that language functions are the responsibility of a specific site or sites. This might seem to be a reasonable conclusion if we were confident that tasks such as generating word lists are representative of a meaningful component of language processing and that we are not just observing the neural site associated with the experimental task.

Despite problems with details, it is now clear that certain language activities can be associated with specific areas of the brain. The results from the Wise et al. study demonstrated that processing single words did provoke activity in the posterior area and that the silent generation of verbs produced additional activity in Broca's area. Beretta's subjects silently generated the regular and irregular forms. So how far are such studies instructive about the relationship between language and neural representation? The field is confusing. Tyler and colleagues discuss and demonstrate a difference between results obtained on-line, for example by reaction times compared with cortical activation. For example, although non-aphasic subjects may be slower to process verbs compared with nouns, or abstract verbs and nouns compared with concrete verbs and nouns, there is no difference (in their studies) in the cortical areas activated during these tasks (Tyler, Russell, Fadili and Moss 2001).

Howard (1997:290), reviewing the evidence from both lesion studies and cerebral blood flow studies, recognises that group studies do show that there is a tendency for specific regions of the brain to be associated with specific language tasks. He reviews a number of studies that report on investigations using imaging, electrical stimulation and monitoring of cerebral blood flow. Ojemann (1994), using a picture-naming task, showed that sites tend to be quite small, that there is considerable individual variation across subjects but that the site involved for the majority of subjects (79 per cent) was in the area traditionally associated with naming. Blood flow studies (such as Wise et al. 1991) also focus on single-word processing. For example, increase in blood flow is monitored while subjects are required either to monitor speech input or to produce lists of words. Subjects listening to real words versus white noise or real words versus nonsense words are found to have greater blood flow activity in the left superior gyrus when listening to real words. Other processing tasks have included monitoring lists of nouns for a specific lexical or semantic category or for words beginning with a specific letter. Production tasks include repetition tasks and tasks which require lists of words to be generated, as for example, generating nouns of a specific semantic category or generating verbs when given a noun. All these tasks are strongly associated with activity in the temporal cortex although tasks involving verb generation also produce activity in the frontal regions.

There are various limitations to these studies. To date, the kinds of tasks given have been limited, partly by the restraints of the equipment used but more especially by the desire to have tasks that will yield information about a specific feature of language as such as the processing of irregular versus regular past-tense verbs. To this end, tasks involving word lists are used. It is difficult to see how the generation of a list of verbs can tell us anything about the computation of verbs within a sentence unless one has the view of language that a sentence comprises only a list of words.

Studies with aphasic subjects

There are a number of studies that have investigated neural sites and neural activity during language tasks using aphasic subjects. As with studies using non-aphasic subjects, the results are open to various interpretations. For example, recordings of event-related brain potentials (ERPs) have been interpreting recruitment of homologous neural areas in subjects with both Broca's and Wernicke's aphasia. Increased brain activity related to certain sentence structures has been interpreted as recruitment of increased processing resources. Reaction times to lexical tasks has been interpreted as evidence that lexical knowledge is not lost in aphasia but that accessing that knowledge is abnormally slow. It would seem that Wernicke's subjects have particular problems with integrating lexical knowledge. This has been interpreted as a problem of slow activation and slow integration rather than a comprehension problem. To date, the number of subjects is small; distinctions may not be made between Broca's and Wernicke's aphasic subjects (Hagoort, Wassenaar and Brown 2003) and interpretations vary. There are a number of excellent examples and reviews of this research in aphasic and non-aphasic subjects (e.g. Hagoort and Kutas 1995, Swaab, Brown and Hagoort 1997, Caplan 2000, Thompson, in press).

Results of this research show that, for normal subjects at least, the temporal region of the brain is associated with tasks involving the generation and the monitoring of nouns and verbs but that the frontal lobe may play a part in verb generation. This comes as no surprise, as it has long been recognised that the generation of nouns is problematic for patients who have sustained lesions in Wernicke's area, while verb generation is difficult for speakers with Wernicke's and Broca's aphasia. This information, based on sophisticated investigations, confirms the claims made by Wernicke based on clinical observation and autopsy results. The individual variation also accords with the consistent finding of variation within the aphasic population. But it would also appear that the lesion data are incompatible with the strong localisation position, although it would be premature to reject the notion that specific parts of the brain are associated with specific language tasks. How far the results on these sorts of tasks are indicative of localised cerebral activity during 'real' spontaneous connected speech remains to be demonstrated.

Summary

In this first chapter fluent aphasia has been introduced and set within the neo-classic framework of syndromes. Brief descriptions of other types of aphasia have been given. We started our study by looking at the work of Wernicke, the neurologist who first described this rather exotic language condition. The descriptions of the syndromes associated with the Boston School followed and the chapter has concluded with a short review of some of the studies that have investigated brain–language relationships. Descriptions of aphasia have changed over the years although much that is written today does not reflect the increased knowledge that is available, and, noticeably, descriptions do not reflect the sophisticated developments made in theoretical linguistics. This is also true of the studies conceived to investigate brain–language relationships. Here we are only at the beginning of what might prove to be the most exciting area of neurolinguistic research.

2 Descriptions of fluent aphasia

I am always TV . . . sometimes . . . I don't care . . . I can't do it . . . it doesn't matter if I can't do it just because I do it but that's all I can because I can't reading.

Introduction

The above quote was the answer given by a fluent aphasic speaker when asked what he did in the evenings. In this chapter we will explore accounts of the speech of fluent aphasia, looking at the characteristics of the language disorder. In particular, we will look at accounts that have attempted to quantify features of the condition and at accounts resulting from a comparison of fluent aphasia and non-fluent aphasia. Some of these accounts result from group studies, although group size is usually small, while others use single cases, following in the tradition of the early aphasiologists such as Wernicke. Some researchers attempt to offer explanations of the phenomena either in terms of psycholinguistic processing or, more unusually, in terms of some linguistic theory of how language is organised. The chapter starts with a brief overview of one model of sentence processing current in cognitive psychology. We then turn to levels of linguistic description, a familiar approach in clinical aphasia in the UK, for our account of production deficits. Comprehension deficits are considered in chapter 6.

A sentence-processing model

Models of language processing are increasingly referred to in the clinical aphasia literature and favoured by cognitive psychologists working in the field. A recent series of papers in *Cognitive Psychology* (2004, volume 21) highlights some of the limitations of the field and, by implication, of models of language processing. (See, for example, papers in this volume by Caplan, Harley and Shalice.) Results of painstaking research using a variety of empirical techniques contradict findings from equally fine research; in a relatively small field of study there are tensions between the advocates of different models; resource-hungry brain studies say little of practical clinical import, as frequently there is little or no correlation between cognitive function and cortical activity (Harley 2000). For example, Tyler and colleagues demonstrate that on-line language tasks may show a difference between processing nouns and verbs or between concrete and abstract words but that this does not correlate with neural activity (Tyler, Russell, Fadili and Moss 2001). Models of single-word processing (e.g. the Psycholinguistic Analysis of Language Processing in Aphasia (PALPA), Kay, Lesser and Coltheart 1992) are used extensively in clinical aphasia in the UK but these will take the clinician only so far, as, sooner or later, many patients require help with sentence construction and comprehension. The single-word processing model has limitations when dealing with language rather than vocabulary, for language production does not proceed by the generation of single words. Linguistics has given us alternative abstract models of sentence structure. Here, words in sentences have hierarchical relationships and these relations differ according to sentence structure. To take a simple example, lexical verbs, such as *see, bake*, may or may not take inflection, depending on the sentence. In the sentences *she bakes a cake, she baked a cake, I bake a cake*, the verbs are finite, that is, inflected. In the diagrammatic representation used in generative grammar, *bake*, *baked* and *bakes* are finite verbs checked, or moved (depending on the model of analysis used) in a node, INF (inflection). In the sentences *I was baking, I like to bake*, the verb bake is not finite and is not in the INF node. This abstract notion has been used to account for the difference found in aphasic speech between the ability to produce finite versus non-finite verbs. Sentence-processing models embrace vocabulary selection, grammar and meaning although, not surprisingly, they remain under-specified at every level (Thompson and Faroqi 2002).

One of the most frequently cited models is Levelt's (1989) which has undergone various developments (e.g. Bock and Levelt 1994, Levelt, Roelofs and Meyer 1999). Levelt's model of sentence processing comprises a series of components or levels, that is, a serial approach to building language. In diagram form, it suggests there are discrete modules but the model is actually conceived as a complex integrated and interactive system. The process of producing a sentence involves conceiving what is to be said (the message level), retrieving lexical items from a mental store and assigning these items grammatical roles (the functional level), ordering constituents of the sentence (the positional planning), inserting inflection and grammatical 'function' words (the positional level) and, finally, phonological encoding.

In this model, the first stage, *the message level*, involves semantic or possible pre-semantic activity. The notion of what is to be expressed is unspecified, for example *to do with people and a gift*. People with aphasia often indicate that they know what they want to say but fail to do so. Stages two and three, the *functional and positional level*, entail grammatical encoding as well as lexical selection. At the *functional level*, lexical items are selected, *mother girl roses give*, and linked with their grammatical roles, *girl-subject, roses-direct object, mother-indirect-object*. Thematic roles (that is, the function of the NPs, who does what to whom) are specified *girl-agent, roses-theme, mother-recipient*. At these stages, words are selected and, although assigned roles, do not yet have their full phonological form. They are known as lemmas and carry grammatical information (word status, noun or verb) and semantic information. It is thought that it is at this stage, the *functional*, that verb lemmas carry semantic information and information about the type of phrase structure needed. So, for example, the verb *bake* comes with the information that it takes two arguments (NPs), one that will do the action of baking and one that will experience that action. Further, the verbs allow various sentence frames: they can act as agentive verbs, as in *I broke a glass* but also as ergative verbs, *the glass broke*.

At the *positional level*, the sentence constituents are ordered. This parallels phrase structure building in the descriptions of the linguistic hierarchical tree structures. In the processing model, the structure is driven by the information contained in the lemmas selected. Bearing in mind the options verbs bring, the 'decision' as to which sentence structure to build – active or passive, or use of verb, agentive or ergative, for example – has already been taken at the *functional level*. It is at the *positional* level that inflection is applied and function words inserted. It is not clear how this happens.

This model provides a modular account that lends itself to thinking about types of aphasic deficits in terms of processes or modules. In specifying different modules involved in production there is an assumption in the aphasia literature that part of the process may be damaged. This allows various phenomena of aphasic output to be 'mapped' onto the model. Deficits may be seen as occurring at the different levels or stages of sentence production, and therapy may be designed to target the assumed processes of the model (Jain 2004). Thompson and Faroqi (2002) give a useful overview of sentence-processing models and how they relate to aphasia.

There is minimal overlap with the framework that will be used in this chapter. In the linguistic description discussed below, retrieval of lexical items and building of the phrase structure of the sentence have some equivalence to the functional and positional levels of the processing model of Levelt. There is also a stage when the sentence constituents receive phonological form, known as *spell out*. This descriptive framework allows for mapping from deficit to linguistic level. This is what we will now explore.

Impairments to a dual language system

The model used throughout this monograph is one where it is assumed that language has two domains, the lexical and the grammatical domain. Lexis is sometimes referred to as the mental lexicon, the mental store or mental dictionary we have of words. The term lexis, rather than word, is used here in order to encompass forms of words such as *boat* and *boats*. Each word has semantic and grammatical information stored with it. This information includes information on word class, distribution restrictions and about which complements or argument structures are required or permitted. Thus the selection of a word, especially a verb, specifies certain dimensions of the intended sentence. For example, a sentence that starts *I hear* needs to proceed either with an adjectival phrase such as *very well*, or if a noun phrase (NP) follows, such as *the bird song*, that NP has to have a semantic feature [+ audible]. A sentence that starts *I feel* needs to proceed with a NP that has a semantic feature [+ tactile] or [+ emotion] such as *very happy*. The verb selected thus contains information about what other constituents are permitted. Each word, or lexical item, in addition to meaning, at some abstract level has phonological form, an abstract representation of the sounds that will eventually be produced. These, in turn, are transformed into speech sounds by the musculature of the sub-vocal, vocal and supra-vocal tract. The associated meanings and sounds of lexical items are referred to as *features* and theses features combine into lexical items.

The second domain, the grammar, is the computational part of language whereby units of the language are combined to form phrases and sentences. Instead of two domains, we could posit three domains, or elements. Chomsky (2000:10) describes language as involving three elements: properties of sound and meaning: that is, (1) *features*; (2) items assembled from these features: that is *lexical items*; (3) *complex expressions* constructed from these 'atomic' units. The computational system has, he continues, two basic operations, firstly assembling the lexical items and secondly forming larger syntactic objects.

These three elements of language are all implicated in aphasia, giving rise to difficulties in the processing of the *form* (or sound) of words, difficulties in processing the *meaning* of words and difficulties with the computational aspect of language, that is marking tense, agreement and forming sentences. Each of these three levels can be impaired. Lexical features of sound and meaning can be differentially impaired, as can computational processes. Operations combining the elements of language to form sentences are more obviously problematic in Broca's aphasia although they are also found in fluent aphasia. The outstanding difficulty in fluent aphasia is that of retrieving lexical items and this difficulty may involve selecting an item with the wrong semantic features or selecting an item where phonological features have been assembled incorrectly, Chomsky's first two elements. Although difficulties in the domain of grammar have not been so readily recognised, this element of language is not entirely spared in fluent aphasia.

The idea that the language faculty comprises a lexicon and computational processes is not an idea confined to one school or one linguistic theory. As Clashen (1999:991) observes, an assumption of a dual system 'does not hinge on the adoption of a particular theory'. His summarised definition of a dual system states that 'the language faculty has a modular structure and consists of two basic components, a lexicon of (structured) entries and a computational system of combined operations to form larger linguistic expressions from lexical entries'. This differs in detail from Chomsky's three-element model where computational processes are involved with the combination of the features that form the lexical items as well as with the combination of the lexical units that form the syntactic elements. Either can be recruited when trying to build a description of aphasia.

The duality of language in which there is a mental lexicon and a computation component has not been influential in the aphasia literature although notions of language as a modular system are commonplace. Models where different modules, or levels of language comprehension and production, may be affected, are pervasive. However, even when discussion of aphasia deficits are linked to the notion of a dual system, there are some fundamental differences in how the lexical and the computational system have been conceptualised and utilised within the study of aphasia. Within this literature, ideas about language owe more to early work by the first aphasiologists and the clinically observed features of Broca's and Wernicke's aphasias than to current linguistic debate.

There are other features of language that fall outside the domains of lexis and grammar, although none of these domains operates in isolation and the different elements or levels of linguistic description (terms that are sometimes used interchangeably) impact on one another in non-aphasic and aphasic speakers. A speaker also has access to pragmatic knowledge and to general knowledge of the world. Both of these domains contribute to the processing of language but there is no convincing evidence that either is separately deficient in aphasia. Pragmatic skills might not function efficiently, but that is because language is deficient. Aphasic speakers retain the knowledge of how to use language. Supra-segmental features also appear to be preserved in fluent aphasia. We will consider two of these, rate of speech and prosody.

We will start by looking at non-segmental features of speech, rate and prosody. Rate of speech is part of the classic description of fluent aphasia; it is said to be rapid, hyper-fluent or excessive in some way. Our data question this view. Characteristics of fluent aphasia speech will then be described under headings that reflect broad levels of linguistic description. We examine errors at the phonological and lexical levels and finally, we discuss the presence of grammatical errors in fluent aphasia.

The so-called 'press of speech'

The nature of the prosody and rate of speech in fluent aphasia is in sharp contrast to that found in Broca's aphasia or agrammatism. Unlike non-fluent speech that is slow and effortful, fluent aphasia seems to have normal prosody and a normal rate of delivery. Some descriptions include 'press of speech' as a characteristic, suggesting that the rate of speech is faster than normal. There is little to say about the prosodic features of fluent aphasia but rate of speech is said to be around 200 words per minute (Benson and Ardila 1996). This, though, is the rate usually given for normal, non-aphasic speech. It therefore appears unremarkable and accounts, in part, for why this speech sounds, from a distance, normal. There is some empirical evidence to support this.

Edwards and Garman (1989) (hereafter E and G) compared the rate of speech of a Wernicke's aphasic speaker (Mr V) with an age-matched control (Mr W). Both subjects were of a comparable age and educational background and were both recently retired from semi-skilled work. Samples of spontaneous speech were collected for analysis. The subjects were invited to talk about the same topic (their previous employment) while the investigator provided minimal input. A number of variables were investigated. On measures of quantity of speech (words per utterance, words per minute and pauses) there was little difference between the aphasic and the non-aphasic speaker. A lack of difference between the speech of control and aphasic subjects or even a slightly slower rate for fluent aphasic speakers has been found in other studies (Bird and Franklin 1996) suggesting that on this measure, speed, there may be little difference between the aphasic and the non-aphasic speaker. So what is 'press of speech'?

There are a couple of explanations why it seems that fluent aphasic speakers, and especially those with Wernicke's aphasia, appear to talk faster and more than non-aphasic speakers, displaying what is sometimes called 'hyperfluency'. The first is related to the structure of conversation that is typical with these speakers. The second, E and G suggest, arises because of the difficulty fluent aphasic speakers have in expressing themselves. In the analysis presented in the E and G study, although the speaker with aphasia spoke at a similar rate to the non-aphasic speaker, there are various indices that distinguish the aphasic and the non-aphasic speaker and illustrate some characteristics of each speaker's connected speech. Caution is needed in the interpretation of these results as the sample was not elicited as a conversation. Each speaker was asked to talk about his previous employment and the person collecting the sample made only a minimal contribution. Nevertheless, two measures that are used as indicators of conversational competence, number of turns and overlaps of speakers' turns, were applied and showed that the aphasic speaker, Mr V was not permitting as much conversational participation as the non-aphasic control, Mr W. Even though the task was to talk about events ('tell me about the work you used to do'), the non-aphasic speaker permitted comments and contributions from his interlocutor to an extent that the aphasic speaker did not. The low number of interventions from the interlocutor when she was with Mr V arose from two main factors that will be familiar to anyone who is used to talking with people with fluent aphasia. First, it is difficult to cut into the stream of speech when the meaning is unclear, for natural conversational boundaries are not clear. Secondly, when the content is incomprehensible it becomes very difficult to contribute anything other than repeated requests for clarification.

The analyses given by E and G show the extent of such difficulties. The number of unintelligible utterances is high in the speech of Mr V compared with those in the non-aphasic speech. The aphasic speaker has a large number of lexical errors, especially in noun slots. Some were omissions and some lexical paraphasia, that is when a word is 'substituted' for the assumed target. Some paraphasic errors involved extra phonemes added to a recognisable stem, for example *week* was frequently pronounced as *weeketh*, where the target word could be easily guessed but in some utterances substitutions occurred and the target word remained unrecognisable. Some of these paraphasic errors took a similar phonemic structure to the ones where the target words were recognisable in that they contained the same nonsense syllable that was added to real words, for example *timeth*, although a possible root *time* made no sense in the discourse. Here there is no way of guessing what

the target was. Given that Mr V had considerable problems with word finding, especially nouns, and that his speech contained a number of neologisms,
it is not surprising that he was difficult to understand and that verbal clashes
resulted. The verbal clashes and overlaps arose as a consequence of the aphasia
while the minimal contribution from the person who was eliciting the sample
may be a consequence of the task. The sample of the non-aphasic speech was
collected in similar circumstances but in this case, because the speaker could
be understood, the therapist was able to contribute occasional comments and
encouragement.

This small study illustrates that, while rate of speech may be normal in
fluent aphasia, the impression of the so-called 'press of speech' may arise
because of failure of the fluent aphasic speaker to maintain normal conversational behaviours. Difficulties with maintaining conversation may be regarded
as part of the aphasic profile arising as a consequence of the aphasia. There are
different views on this. In my experience it is neither accurate nor helpful to
regard conversational skills as 'impaired' in fluent aphasia. These speakers are
able to display all other types of appropriate conversational behaviour such as
giving and receiving greetings, participating in leave-taking routines, request-
ing, thanking and showing awareness of the need to respond to questions. The
inability or reduced ability to answer questions, or indeed to ask questions
appropriately, to repair conversational breakdowns or to maintain topics within
conversations is, in my experience, a consequence of the language disorder
rather than part of it.

Deficits in the lexical domain

Although rate and prosody are normal in fluent aphasic speech, it doesn't take
long before it becomes apparent to the listener that the speech is abnormal, often
meaningless, as in the example given at the beginning of this chapter. In the most
severe case, it may be entirely meaningless, as can be seen from examples given
in the previous chapter. Loss or difficulties in meaning arise, primarily, as a result
of lexical errors that are often cited as the most striking characteristic of fluent
aphasia (Benson and Ardila 1996). Davis (2000:37) suggests that the existence
of lexical difficulties and the preservation of 'recognisable sentence structure'
in Wernicke's aphasia are 'indicative of a dissociation of word-finding from
fundamental syntactic construction'. This notion of dissociation of vocabulary
and structure is pervasive throughout the aphasic literature and may be seen to
be in tune with the notion of the dual nature of language, the two domains of
the language faculty.

Phonological and lexical paraphasias

Lexical features may be damaged although on-line studies suggest that the actual store of lexical items is intact. Nevertheless, off-line, there are errors in the form and meaning of words, both of which are known as paraphasias. Fluent aphasic speakers, especially those with conduction aphasia, make many errors of word form, which are considered and described as phonological errors. Some errors involve incorrect selection of individual phonemes within a word and are known as phonemic paraphasias. (In the Boston terminology they are, confusingly, known as literal paraphasia.) Such errors can be observed most readily when the substitution of an *incorrect* phoneme does not interfere with the recognition of the target word. So, for example, *tog* may be produced instead of *dog*, and provided that the target word is recognised, as for example, in the sentence *I took my tog for a walk last night* or in a picture description task, then meaning is not necessarily compromised. Errors may be related to the target along phonemic dimensions, as in the example above where the relationship of manner and place of production is preserved while voicing is at variance. But the target is not always as apparent as in the example above. It may be difficult to decide, or impossible to decide, whether the error is one of phonemic substitution or whether a whole word has been substituted, as a phonemic substitution may lead to a real word, rather than to a non-word. If the initial phoneme in *chair* is replaced by /f/, for example, then the result is a real word. When conducting error analysis it is important to have enough data to enable such possibilities to be considered.

There is some debate in the literature as to why or where phonological errors are generated. Some attempts have been made to compare sound errors made by aphasic speakers with 'slips of the tongue' made by non-aphasic speakers. In non-aphasic speech phonemic errors are thought to be anticipatory, that is, the sound produced in error is one that is produced later downstream or is said to be perseverative, that is, a sound previously used is repeated erroneously. Continuous speech data from speakers with Wernicke's aphasia has been examined in various studies, and whether anticipatory errors predominate in aphasic speech, as in non-aphasic speech, is rather inconclusive, as results vary according to methodology. One reason is that it is difficult to get agreement among investigators about the intended target and hence to decide whether an error is anticipatory or perseverative. Agreement may be as low as 34 per cent. Further, identification of context in which errors should be judged can vary especially if frequency of phoneme use is taken into consideration. There is also variation in the frequency of error types depending on the severity of the Wernicke's aphasia, leading to varying quantities of data being eliminated from these kinds of analyses (Goldman, Schwartz and Wiltshire 2001). These researchers found both types of errors, with a tendency for word-initial position, to be influential. The existence of anticipatory errors in Wernicke's aphasia is evidence that the speaker has some kind of lexical plan while the existence of preservative errors suggests that there may be a problem with clearing the phonological loop within short-term memory.

Substitution of a whole word is referred to as a lexical paraphasia and can take various forms. A lexical paraphasia may be interpreted as a 'semantic disruption' that is, some kind of disturbance to the relationship between form and meaning. The aphasic speaker is thought to have lost or to have intermittent or faulty access to the meaning of words. S/he can no longer reliably make an accurate selection between semantically related words within the mental lexicon and hence produces errors. This type of deficit is identified by the types of errors made and by performance on certain tasks. Typically such speakers will fail tasks such as:

- categorising words, for example sorting the words *apple, car, bus, pear, taxi, strawberry* into the categories of *fruit* and *vehicles*;
- judging which word in a group of words, such as *chair, bed, table, cloud, cupboard* is unrelated, semantically, to the other group members;
- judging the semantic relatedness of words such as *argue* and *row*; *grow* and *shoot* (Martin and Blossom-Stach 1986).

The fact that some lexical errors are semantically related to the target word may signify a disrupted semantic system. It is assumed that the speaker has some kind of mental representation of the target word but is unable to select the lexical item with sufficient precision and therefore selects one that is incorrect although semantically related, sometimes described as a semantic neighbour. The selection may result in a word that is close in meaning, for example, *boy* for *nephew*, but semantic relatedness does not always produce a word close in meaning. For example, the use of *man* for *wife*, which one of my patients frequently used, leads to confusion even though these words share the semantic features [+ animate], [+ human] and [+ adult]. Crucially, they do not share the semantic features of [+ female] and [+ close relation]. We can interpret this kind of error as a disruption to feature selection. It has been described as an equal activation of neighbours whereas what is required is for the target word to have superior activation in order to be selected. However, when a speaker regularly uses a substitution, as, in the example above, *man* for *wife*, then it cannot be that this error arises because of the equal activation of lexical neighbours. In these cases, the substitution – in our example, *man* – must be regularly receiving superior activation over *wife*. Such examples are infrequent in fluent aphasia and may not be observed in experimental conditions but are observed by clinicians who get to know their patients over many weeks or months.

When an incorrect word is accessed, it may be clear that it is not the target word but, despite a semantic association, the intended meaning of the speaker may still be obscure. So in the utterance

(1)   *I couldn't hear the pain*

although *pain* is a real word it doesn't have the necessary feature required by the verb *hear*. This verb requires the following NP to have the semantic feature of noise, something that can be heard. *Pain* cannot be heard, putting aside poetic genre here. So either the verb or the noun in this sentence must be incorrect. It was not possible, in this instance, to guess which word was the target word. The speaker was talking about the onset of aphasia and maybe he was trying to describe how he couldn't understand. On the other hand, he may have switched topics at this point and have been referring to his physical condition and the fact that he wasn't in pain. If *hear* was the intended verb then he needed a different noun. If the noun, *the pain*, was correct, then he needed a different verb. Both *feel* and *hear* have the same predicate argument structure, each verb takes an obligatory argument after the verb. So in this example, the syntactic structure is correct. Additionally, the substituted word, whichever it may be, fulfils the requirements of word class: either we have a verb-verb substitution or a noun-noun substitution.

However, although the substitution satisfies the grammatical requirements of argument structure it does not satisfy its semantic requirements. As a result, meaning is faulty although structure is not. This is a good exemplar of an error that can be classified as a problem with meaning rather than with grammar. Had, however, the two verbs required different argument structures, if, for example, the substituted verb had been *put* instead of *hear*, then the argument structure would have been violated because the verb *put* requires three, not two, arguments. So if the speaker had said

(2)   *I couldn't put the pain*

then neither the meaning nor the structure requirements of the verb arguments would have been met.

There is a tendency for lexical substitutions to come from the same grammatical class, but argument structure is not always preserved. Here is an example of a noun-noun substitution taken from some continuous speech data where the task was to retell the Noah's Ark story.

(3)   *Noah, he went into the barn . . . in . . . went . . . in into the sea*

In example (3) because of shared knowledge of the Noah's Ark story and because the hesitations signal some lexical retrieval problems, we are able to make certain assumptions about lexical substitutions. First we might assume that *barn* is a lexical paraphasic error replacing *ark*. There are semantic associations in that both a *barn* and an *ark* are buildings capable of being dwellings: they share certain semantic features. This substitution is followed by a phrase where the speaker attempts, we can assume, to correct *the barn* but actually produces *the sea* instead of *the ark*. *The sea* is clearly associated with the watery context of the Noah's Ark story but it doesn't fit into this sentence. However, if *the sea* is a substitution for *ark* then it shares some similar semantic features. The ark floats on water and shares [+ water] with *sea*. Of course, we can't be sure of the speaker's intended target but it is likely that the errors here reflect some kind of semantic association, although the association is with more than one target. These types of lexical paraphasias, if related in meaning in some way, are also called semantic lexical paraphasic errors. The terminology used by Goodglass and colleagues differs. They refer to such errors as 'verbal' paraphasic errors.

Explanations of these sorts of paraphasias involve notions of the lexicon being organised, in some abstract way, with words which are similar in meaning, or related in meaning in some way, stored as near neighbours. Thus even erroneous retrieval is not entirely random but just not accurate enough to select the desired target word: a 'near neighbour' gets selected. However, it could be that the aphasic speaker, aware of the inability to retrieve the desired lexical item at that point chooses the lexical item nearest to the intended target. Maybe such episodes resemble experiences of healthy non-native speakers, who, unable to provide the required word in their second (or third) language, supply the best available word. The speaker may know it isn't right but it is an available word nearest in meaning. When listening to speakers with fluent aphasia, each of these accounts seems plausible. Sometimes, the speakers clearly know that the word is wrong and indicate so and may struggle to correct the error, but, at other times, they may seemed resigned to the fact that this is the closest match. Often, however, speakers with Wernicke's aphasia are not aware of their errors, especially in the early stages, or indeed for some years after becoming aphasic, if the condition is severe. In this case, aphasic speakers will not struggle to retrieve the correct word but continue with long monologues, sometimes becoming agitated when they realise that their interlocutor cannot understand them.

The fact that these two types of errors, errors of phoneme selection and errors of word selection, can occur separately in aphasia illustrates how features of sound and meaning can be differentially impaired. These different types of errors are cited as two separate stages of production of words, one the specification of the lexical item and the second the phonemic stage where phonemes of a word are assembled ready to be converted to phonetic specification and eventually to the articulatory processes. In cases where the paraphasic substitution may be related, phonemically or lexically, to the target word, it is assumed that the speaker has some concept of the target word. If the error is semantically related, as in examples (2) and (3) above, then it is assumed that there is some kind of mental representation of the target word. Grammatical status may or may not be correct (we have seen how nouns are substituted for nouns) but meaning is not correctly specified. If the error is considered to be one of phonemic selection, then it is assumed that the word has been fully specified in terms of meaning and grammatical class, but phonological specification is faulty. It has also been assumed that there may be a combination of errors where a word is mis-selected at the lexical level and then incorrect phonemes are selected at the phonemic level. This is given as some type of explanation for lexical paraphasic errors that seem to be unrelated to the target word. Where strings of non-words are produced with normal intonation, as is the case of severe Wernicke's aphasia, the output is known as jargon aphasia and a case has been made that in severe cases of aphasia, non-words may be a some kind of random output from the phonological store.

Attempts have been made to make categorical distinctions between these types of paraphasias, phonemic and lexical, and to link them with different syndromes. Thus, phonemic errors characterise conduction aphasia and lexical errors, that is, ones involving a whole word, characterise Wernicke's aphasia. In reality, patients often show both types of error and, furthermore, it may be difficult to decide whether an error is phonemic or lexical. These two types of paraphasias can be further subdivided depending on what is thought to be the underlying processing deficit or where within speech production process the deficit is located. Some aphasiologists use a psycholinguistic rather than a linguistic model. Such models of language processing propose steps or components of processing, an assumed non-linguistic cognitive activity. These models are better specified for single-word production than for sentence production but none is very detailed. The models contain stages or components that correspond in a loose way to the elements of language we discussed at the beginning of this chapter. Phonemic and semantic components are identified, but in addition some form of processing – a short-term memory, working memory or phonological loop – is also invoked to account for errors found in aphasic speech. These are useful in that they can help sort out the components of lexical errors but offer very little in terms of understanding sentence deficits or how words are produced within sentences.

Although in off-line studies it appears that the problem lies with lexical access, on-line studies have suggested that lexical items can be accessed but that access is slow. To date, most of these studies have looked at processing and comprehension rather than production but there are likely to be advances in the coming years that may completely change our view of how these errors occur.

Non-linguistic variable in lexical access

Words vary by more than form, meaning and grammatical class. They vary in frequency, familiarity and, it is claimed, age of acquisition and imageability. Words also vary in phonological complexity, length and other factors. Testing for the effect of these variables on lexical recall in aphasia, including fluent aphasia, has produced mixed results, partly, it is suspected, because of the procedures used. First, frequency has, in the past, been based on corpora of written data, such as Francis and Kucera (1982), and it is now accepted that frequency scores for written data probably vary compared with those obtained for spoken data. To date, the corpora of spoken data are smaller and may not be representative of the speech of the subjects under review. Familiarity, age of acquisition and imageability scores are devised by listener judgement where the number of subjects making the judgements is relatively small. Not surprisingly, there is a high correlation between familiarity and age of acquisition scores although most work has been on nouns.

These factors can be shown to have an effect, but not on all subjects, a fact that is clinically as well as theoretically important. For example, Davidoff and Masterson (1996) found that age of acquisition was associated with errors for only four of their eleven subjects, but age of acquisition and imageability for some of the four (number not specified). They found that three of their six variables, frequency, imageability and visual complexity, never predicted errors of naming in their study whereas age of acquisition, name agreement and familiarity predicted errors in some of their subjects. Berndt and her colleagues had similar findings for accessing of verbs. Comparing the ability to access verbs and nouns, she found that grammatical class was a much stronger influence on word access than other factors, such as frequency.

Examples of paraphasic errors

Davis (2000:84) briefly discusses whether lexical errors can be thought of as semantic errors or whether they should more accurately be thought of as deficits of lexical access. He reviews some work that has examined aphasic subjects' ability, for example, to make rapid decisions about categorical relationships between words. The results that he quotes make it clear that lexical accessing problems are not always associated with deficits in the semantic system. It is true that patients will often indicate that they know a name of an object and will reject inaccurate names but still fail to produce the correct names. Trying to decide the origins of a lexical error can only be a matter of speculation, as these examples illustrate. They are taken from a subsection of the Boston Diagnostic Aphasia Examination (Goodglass and Kaplan 1983). In examples (4) and (5) the aphasic speaker was attempting to name pictures of objects.

	Target	*Response*
(4)	key	door
(5)	ear	eyes

In these examples we can see that the speaker knew something about the target. Although not able to access the target word, in each case he produced a word within the noun category. In the following examples, the speaker was answering questions from the Boston Diagnostic Aphasia Examination (Goodglass and Kaplan 1983). In this section, the patient has to understand the question and provide, depending on the question, a noun or verb.

(6)	What do you do with soap?	water
(7)	What do you do with a pencil?	reading
(8)	What do we cut paper with?	not a knife, it's a . . .
(9)	How many things in a dozen?	one

The first two examples above demonstrate that the speaker knew something about the target answer. Although not able to produce the correct verb, the answers, *water* and *reading* are semantically related to the target verbs *wash* and *write/draw*. Here, we see one error that crosses grammatical word categories, (*water* (noun) substituted for *wash* (verb)) and one that is within the category (*reading* and *draw* are both verbs). In example (8) it would seem that again the speaker has an awareness of the intended target; he produces the name of an object, *knife*, which shares certain semantic features, also cuts. In example (9) it may be the final word (a noun of number) that triggers the response rather than a search for the target verb. Alternatively, he may not understand this, or indeed the other questions. What he might be doing is to produce a word associated with the noun carrying the major nuclear stress in the question. An argument against this interpretation is that he shows, in example (8) at least, that he is aware that his response is incorrect. There may be a number of different reasons involved here.

Semantic associations between intended target and lexical substitution may be found especially if the sentence structure is intact. Guessing the intended target may be more problematic when sentence structure is faulty. For example, when a speaker says

(10)   *two weeks, two weeks today I'm going in a doctor doctor on the twenty-sixth of July*

we may be able to guess that he is talking about some kind of medical appointment but be unable to guess the exact details. In this example, there are several possible reconstructions that would be plausible. It may be that there is a noun-noun substitute, *doctor* for *hospital*, in which case the determiner *a* is misplaced. Whereas *doctor* requires an indefinite article, *hospital* does not, unless a specific hospital is being denoted. If the existence of the determiner *a* indicates that a noun phrase is to follow *in*, then the noun phrase should be *hospital* rather than *doctor*. If, however, he is to see a doctor, then either there is a verb missing, such as *to see*, or, minimally, there is an incorrect preposition *in* instead of *to*. However, this would give us *I'm going to a doctor on the twenty-sixth of July*: still rather an odd sentence for British English. We might expect *I'm going to the doctor's* if he is talking about his regular doctor or, if not, *I'm going to see a doctor* if the identity of the doctor is unknown or unspecified by the speaker. If, however, he is talking about an out-patient appointment at a hospital (which I think he was), then the sentence should have been *I'm going to hospital* not *in hospital*. If he was to be admitted to hospital, then we would expect something like *I'm going into hospital on the twenty-sixth of July*. And there are probably other possible reconstructions. As it stands, the sentence is neither grammatical nor semantically intact. We do not know what message the speaker is trying to convey as the message is obscured by a variety of lexical problems. Not only is the selection of prepositions, determiners and nouns problematic but, once selected, these lexical items do not come with appropriate arguments. The resulting sentence is one that is grammatically and semantically unacceptable.

These examples exemplify errors where we have assumed that some kind of substitution or omission has taken place. Sometimes the omission of words is more transparent because of the preceding sentence as in (11) and (12) below where (11) gives meaning to *couldn't nothing*:

(11)   *I could walk quite quick on me foot one foot is a bit at night*

(12)   *I couldn't nothing*

In (11) part of the NP (*is a bit*) is missing and in (12) part of the VP is missing. In both these examples, the omission interferes with the meaning of the utterance, illustrating the notion that what is faulty in fluent aphasia affects meaning even if the deficit does not originate in the semantic domain. In (11) the speaker is unable to describe what is wrong with his foot and in (12) the omission of the lexical verb compromises the meaning of the sentence.

Lexical paraphasia, word class and sentence construction

As we have seen, substitutions may be within category, *doctor/hospital to/in*, but this is not always the case. One fluent aphasic speaker has, for years, described his aphasia as

(13)   *I know it but I just can't sentence it.*

where *sentence* is used as a verb although we can be almost sure that the homophone *sentence* as a verb is not the intended target word. It isn't clear whether within-class substitutions are really more common or whether they are just easier to identify. Problems with word selection can affect all types of words, as illustrated above, and it is the pervasive nature of the difficulty that casts some doubt on whether the notion of semantic disruption is a sufficient explanation for the lexical paraphasias observed in fluent aphasia. Indeed, substitution of closed-class words would not be characterised as a symptom of a semantic deficit, yet it is an essential feature of paragrammatism: 'paragrammatism is marked by the substitution . . . of function words and grammatical morphemes' (Martin and Blossom-Stach 1986:197) and separates Wernicke's and conduction aphasia from anomia, where the main deficit is difficulty in accessing open-class words, most commonly, nouns. Martin and Blossom-Stach noted that although semantic disruption might account for problems with content words, they queried whether the notion of semantic disruption provides an adequate explanation for the problems with the selection of function words.

   In fluent aphasia there is often a high proportion of incomplete sentences as in (14):

(14)   *and then I was . . .*

(15)   *the next day I felt a bit ill*

where the speaker is unable to complete the sentence in (14) and restarts in (15) using a reformulated sentence and a different verb. It is hard to explain why the speaker was unable to complete the sentence in example (14) with *ill* and yet was able to use it in (15). Examples such as this give rise to a whole raft of possible explanations. Firstly, the success on the second attempt may suggest that the problem is, at least in part, one of slow access to the lexicon rather than loss of lexical items, it takes time to access *ill*. The word was not accessed in time to complete (14) but was available for the second attempt (15). Secondly, using a different verb, one with more semantic associations, the speaker succeeds in producing a grammatically correct and semantically plausible sentence. If this is the case, is there some self-priming, semantically based operation that can occasionally kick in? The copular verb requires an adjective complement in this sentence as does *felt*. How is it that the speaker is unable to access *ill* but can, within seconds, access *a bit ill*? In both sentence frames *ill* would be considered an open-class word; so one cannot argue, in this case, that word class is an influence. Finally (although the reader may well think of yet more possible explanations), an explanation might rest on a different assumption altogether. It may be that this is not, in fact, a failure of word selection but an example of intact, and indeed careful, monitoring. Maybe the speaker recognised that there was a subtle difference in meaning between *being ill* and *feeling ill*, where the latter is often a less severe condition than the former. He may have wished to convey that he felt ill rather than had an illness. Whatever the motivation, he restructured his sentence.

Looking at such examples, collected from spontaneous speech data and naming exercises, we can see that the responses, while generating speculation, do not reveal why such errors occur. There are too many possible explanations. However, analysis of errors occurring in spontaneous speech is a good way of looking at how errors occur in everyday speech. Butterworth and Howard (1987:15) analysed an extensive database comprising spontaneous speech samples collected from four non-aphasic and five fluent aphasic speakers. Their analyses were based on large samples of spontaneous speech, not less than 1,300 words from each of their five subjects and a total of over 12,000 words from the four controls. It may be important to note that their subjects would seem to have moderate to mild aphasic symptoms and so we cannot be confident that their findings would hold for those with more severe fluent aphasia.

Their analysis was motivated by a desire to investigate the nature of para-grammatism in fluent aphasia. In order to do this, they examined all errors in the data, many of which, not surprisingly, were lexical errors. They found lexical errors in both closed-class and open-class words. All closed-class word substitutions were what they call 'within category', that is, the speakers did not substitute a closed-class word with an open-class word but a closed-class with a closed-class word. Open-class word errors were more common but they found that all their five subjects made at least one closed-class error as in the following.

(16)   *they're not prepared to be of helpful*
(17)   *I want everything to be so talk*

Similar errors were found in the control data but with far less frequency (Butterworth and Howard 1987:13).

A grammatical deficit?

We have seen in the above section how lexical problems have consequences for sentence structure. But do ill-formed sentences arise only as a result of lexical difficulties? *Paragrammatism* denotes some 'mismanagement of grammar' but what is '*grammar*'? When aphasiologists talk about 'grammar' they are not necessarily sharing the same concept of grammar as that conceived by Chomsky and other linguists working within a framework of generative grammar. In aphasiology, 'grammar' usually denotes the phenomena of sentence structure, such as verb inflection as well as the relationship between sentence constituents, possibly including the constraints of complement and argument structure. Some researchers look for underlying relationships between sentence constituents, while others describe the surface forms. What these descriptions do not usually address is whether the phenomena observed are evidence of damage to the *grammar* conceptualised as a mental organ by generative linguists, or whether they signify a less central deficit. It is not clear whether what has been described in the literature is a defective grammar (i.e defective or malfunctioning rules and representations), or whether the grammar remains intact but other cognitive processes that implement the grammar are the locus of the deficit. Errors of sentence structure, verb inflection, agreement and so on may be seen not as a grammatical deficit per se but as evidence that there are processing difficulties or even as the result of difficulties in lexical access as shown in the following:

(18)   fox saw the, um, this is awful, what's the name of the animal, uh the dog (doog), holding, uh, the piece of meat

Heard in a continuous stream, it was difficult to follow what the speaker was saying although he was retelling one of Aesop's tales as part of a Boston assessment. However, if we segment this utterance for analysis, we can see that a legitimate sentence structure was interrupted by searching for a lexical item.

(19)   fox saw the (um)

(20)   this is awful

(21)   what's the name of the animal

(22)   (uh) the dog (doog)

(23)   holding (uh) the piece of meat

It looks as though the speaker is able to hang onto the original sentence plan despite commenting on his own performance. (The missing word is *crow* not *dog*.)

Do lexical and sentential errors result from a loss of control?

While there have been controversial claims about whether loss of certain grammatical processes in agrammatism is a loss of representation rather than a processing error, the errors found in fluent aphasia have not excited the same level of scrutiny and debate. On the whole, opinions converge on the notion that, even when errors occur which resemble those in agrammatism, the main deficit is one of lexical access, although not all share this view. Butterworth and Howard (1989:2; hereafter B and H) held the common view that what appear to be syntactic errors are lexical: '[t]he appearance of incorrect syntactic structure can come about by the presence of, say, a noun in place of an adjective or the wrong inflected form of a verb, both of which may be the result of an error in lexical selection.' They conclude their study with a non-linguistic explanation of paragrammatism, maintaining that paragrammatism (and hence the errors they log under each of their categories) is neither a lexical nor a syntactic deficit but a deficit of something involving a 'control mechanism', presumably some kind of cognitive but non-verbal process. Is their conclusion sustainable?

In their study, B and H identified five different types of errors that they classified as paragrammatic errors. They included omission and substitution of open- and closed-class words, inflectional errors and what they called 'constructional errors'. (They also had a 'residue' category.) They defined constructional errors as 'where the order of words or other determinable grammatical process yielded an ungrammatical sentence' (p. 11). These errors were described by the authors as being the 'most striking paragrammatisms' and result from errors in the '*process of constructing the sentence*' rather than from errors of lexical selection or inflection (p. 19). If fluent aphasic speakers have grammatical problems, then these kinds of errors, along with inflectional errors, would be important evidence and worth examining here. The authors divided the category of 'constructional errors' into various subcategories.

Butterworth and Howard had four types of constructional errors: (a) sentence blends; (b) tag errors; (c) illegal NPs in relative clause gaps; (d) pronoun-headed relative clause in object position. Examples from aphasic data are given as follows:

(a) sentence blends:
I'm very want it; presumably blending *I want it* with *I'm very keen on it*

(b) tag errors:
he likes swimming didn't he
but it's silly, aren't they

(c) illegal NPs in relative gaps:
there's one works for a person which is the governor which he has a lot of people work for them. (Although they do not explain which NP is illegal: presumably they are assuming *he* is illegal although *which* should have been *who*.)

(d) pronoun-headed relative clause in object position:
and I'm only just returned it that happened to me

Unfortunately, they also give examples from non-aphasic speech. For example, for 'a pronoun-headed relative clause in object position' *she was talking about power games being played where she worked. The woman there was very jealous of her who was new in the office.* Without intonation information, it is difficult to see what is at fault here. The use of *her who was in the office* seems to be a similar sort of utterance to *she who must be obeyed* and thus somewhat different in status, as far as management of grammar is concerned, from the utterance used by the aphasic speaker. It is not clear whether similar errors did occur in the non-aphasic data.

Constructional errors are reported to have accounted for 15 per cent of the aphasic speakers' paragrammatisms although no quantitative data are given for different categories or for individual subjects. There were a total of 226 (or 20.5 per 1,000 words) paragrammatic errors for the group (p. 11). We can calculate that the group made 34 paragrammatic errors, with a mean of 6.5 per speaker, although we have no way of knowing how consistently errors were spread across subjects.

The type of error that accounts for the largest proportion of paragrammatisms in B and H's data is what they log as *inflexional*. They found a range of what they called inflectional errors in the speech of their five subjects with fluent aphasia but also errors in the speech of the four controls. They give examples of errors of inflection on well-formed words such as *the one mice ran away* (which is not an inflectional error) and *he's went to picks the* as well as inflections on neologisms, although here interpretation is difficult, as illustrated by their examples. The authors found that inflectional errors accounted for 26 per cent of the aphasic speakers' paragrammatic errors and, strangely, 21 per cent of the errors made by their control speakers. They identify nine so-called inflectional errors in the control corpus of 12,644 words and fifty-six in the aphasic corpus of 10,829 words. It is possible that at least some dialectal differences in inflectional morphology (rather than 'slips of the tongue') were tagged as errors in the control data.

The issue is whether the aphasic errors can be considered normal slips of the tongue or whether the frequency of these errors exceeds what we can find in non-aphasic speakers and can be regarded as part of fluent aphasic phenomena. If inflectional errors are indeed the most common type of fluent aphasic error then clearly some deficit in the process of inflection, however that might be conceived, has to be recognised as a defining feature of fluent aphasia. This would run contrary to most work prior to this study. In this study, the errors were distributed as follows: inflectional errors 26 per cent; sentence structure 15 per cent; closed-class words 15 per cent; open-class words 21 per cent.

The data reveal that a considerable proportion (41 per cent) of all paragrammatic errors involved sentence construction or inflection, errors we might consider grammatical, while errors involving open-class words amounted to 21 per cent of the paragrammatic errors. The types of errors found lead the authors to claim that '[a]ll the features considered characteristic of "agrammatism" are found in these patients' (p. 34). However, notwithstanding these findings, the authors rule out any involvement of grammar, saying that there is little support that paragrammatism arises as 'a consequence of some permanent loss or corruption of grammatical rules or grammatical knowledge' (p. 26).

Paragrammatism is, in their view, a deficit of a 'control system' where the 'control system' monitors the modular semantic, lexical, prosodic, phonological and phonetic systems, but not the syntactic system. The claim is that this explanation accommodates both the finding of similar errors in their aphasic and control data. They observe that only the frequency differed between the two groups: speakers had a transient malfunctioning of the system rather than a permanent one. In contrast to the control speakers, the aphasic speakers fail to check output and thus allow errors to be produced that the normally functioning system would filter.

An alternative explanation would be that the grammar, while not permanently lost or corrupted, is damaged in that it functions intermittently. Aphasia has changed the grammar in that it allows more errors through. This explanation sounds very similar to B and H's control mechanism, but the important difference is whether this 'control' is a cognitive process outside the language system or whether it can more reasonably be regarded as part of it. In a version of generative grammar, the Minimalist Program, an operation known as checking checks features of words selected from the mental lexicon. If the features are appropriately checked, the item merges to become part of the nodes and branches of the sentence structure. If features are not correct, then the item crashes. The sentence is not produced. Presumably, in aphasia, the operation of checking does not work efficiently and allows illegal items through. See Arabatzi and Edwards (2002) for a brief description of some agrammatic data using this model.

The one error type that the authors say cannot be accounted for by their control hypothesis is that involving a relative clause that has, illegally, a pronoun in head position. If these occur, and it is not clear from the examples given that they do, then the aphasic speakers are violating grammatical rules. Now the authors have claimed that their data do not support the notion that paragrammatism involves 'permanent loss or corruption of grammatical knowledge' and, in as far as we can judge the data, this would seem to be the case. However, there does seem to be evidence here that these speakers have problems with sentence construction and with verb inflection, which are both part of the grammatical system.

The picture of paragrammatism emerging from this study is one that involves lexical errors, inflectional errors and ill-formed sentences. Can this disorder, then, be viewed as one of deficient lexical processing? Butterworth and Howard dismiss this explanation with rather strange reasoning. They predicted that if the disorder is one primarily of lexical selection then two features should be found. Firstly, they predicted that the lexical selection errors would mainly involve open-class words and, secondly, that the frequency of lexical errors would correlate with the frequency of neologisms. What they found was that the selection of closed-class words was as impaired as the selection of open-class words and that a high number of neologisms did not predict a high number of lexical selection errors. It is difficult to see the logic of these predictions, but the conclusion that paragrammatism cannot be accounted for by the lexical selection errors is in line with other studies. We now turn to grammatical errors.

Grammatical errors

It is commonly observed that fluent aphasic speakers make errors in sentence construction. When expected to produce a picture description as in (24) one fluent aphasic speaker was unable to produce a well-formed sentence (25), although he clearly understood the task and the picture.

(24)   *the monkey is eating the banana*

(25)   the apple . . . /egi/ . . . the bird . . . the monkey . . . monkey eating

In this example there is no auxiliary verb and therefore no tense marked, but the speaker has produced the correct NP in agent position. But errors in assigning the correct thematic role to the sentence NPs is not always achieved (27). The target response is given in (26).

(26)   the dog is biting the cat

(27)   the dog is biting by a baby . . . . no a cat

In this last example, it is not clear whether the speaker knows which of the verb's arguments, *the cat* or *the dog* is the agent and which is the theme. It could be that the search for the correct lexical item, *cat* rather than *baby*, impacts on the ability to form a sentence. Alternatively, the inability to form a grammatical sentence might result from a failed effort to use the passive structure. Whether we can view these sentences as examples of grammatical errors arising from problems with the computational level of language that are independent of the lexical errors is debatable. Each of these examples involves lexical errors as well as grammatical ones and it could be argued that the extra resources required for lexical searching reduce the cognitive resources that are available for computation and thus syntactic errors arise. As syntax is relatively intact in fluent aphasia, compared with non-fluent aphasia, the allocation of resources as an explanation is attractive.

There are several studies that have compared so-called grammatical errors in fluent and non-fluent aphasic speakers. All investigations are, of course, biased by the assumptions the investigators have about the nature of the grammar, and the methodology reflects these assumptions. Even an acknowledgement of this fact does not necessarily lead to authors' explicitly stating their theoretical motivation. Goodglass, Christiansen and Gallagher (1993), while making a similar observation, proceeded to investigate a hotchpotch of grammatical features in fluent and non-fluent aphasic speech. They examined the use of a set of grammatical features in sentence-completion tasks and in free narratives. The seven non-fluent subjects were agrammatic Broca's aphasic speakers and the fluent were seven speakers with conduction aphasia. The sentence-completion tests elicited two types of noun morphology, plural and possessive, and five types of verb morphology: third person singular, tense, auxiliary verb, low content main verb, auxiliary plus complement. Additionally the sentences elicited active voice and passive voice. They found that, while all subjects made errors of both omission and substitution, the fluent aphasic speakers were significantly better at using possessive noun morphology, third person singular marking on verbs and auxiliary verbs in constructions. The example given of an elicitation task actually involves ellipsis of the lexical verb – *these deer are not drinking but this deer* – as well as verb morphology, so errors on this task would not necessarily indicate problems with verb morphology in other contexts.

The authors consider whether the lack of semantic content of the grammatical morphemes contributes to the agrammatic speakers' difficulties. On the assumption that there is, for the agrammatic speakers, 'some inadequacy in the activation of the syntactic frame' (p. 399), the authors surmise that accessing of the required morphemes via a semantic route is not available; thus morphemes are randomly selected. The discussion here does not include consideration of why similar errors are found in the fluent aphasic speech. Presumably, fluent aphasic speakers would not be required to access these morphemes via their semantic route if their syntax representation was intact. Why, then, do they make similar errors?

Errors of inflection were found in data collected from German speakers with fluent aphasia. Kolk and Heeschen (1992) investigated errors of omission and substitution of function words and verb inflection in contrasting tasks. They found that the speakers with Wernicke's aphasia made significantly more substitution errors involving both function words and verb inflection than did the speakers with Broca's aphasia. Both types of aphasic speakers omitted verb inflections although these types of errors were rare for both groups. So, here again, we have evidence that the predominant error type is one of lexical substitution but the fact that inflectional errors described as omission do occur must be noted. Kolk and Heeschen suggest that these two types of aphasia are basically the same. The different manifestation comes about because speakers with Broca's aphasia adopt strategies to cope with the deficit, unlike speakers with Wernicke's aphasia. They suggest that therefore 'paragrammatic output . . . reflects the underlying impairment' (p. 95).

There are problems with this interpretation, not least that it would seem that their Wernicke's aphasic speakers actually made fewer errors than the speakers with Broca's aphasia. It is not possible to confirm this, as raw scores are not given, but the authors do suggest throughout that an incorrect interpretation would be that the speakers with Wernicke's aphasia had a milder form of aphasia (e.g. p. 106). The strategy suggested is that the speakers with Broca's aphasia abandon attempts at sentence structure and utilise ellipsis. In contrast, the Wernicke's aphasic speakers do not employ this strategy, but attempt to use full sentences and hence make errors. Unfortunately, on the task where the Broca's aphasic speakers' production of function words improved, the speakers with Wernicke's aphasia had more omissions. However, rate of omission in the spontaneous speech of the Broca's aphasics increased. It is spontaneous speech where the strategy is supposed to be employed – a strange strategy.

There is further evidence of inflectional errors in fluent aphasia in a study by Bird and Franklin (1996). Samples of spontaneous speech were analysed using Saffran, Berndt and Schwartz's 1989 methodology that results in various indices including an inflection index and an elaboration index. We are told that the errors of these speakers' were within the normal range although the scores given suggest that one subject, DrO, at the second and third time of testing was scoring 0.78 and 0.89 on the inflection index where the normal speakers scored 0.99. Of course, scores of that magnitude also demonstrate that inflection was correct most of the time. Furthermore, at time 1, two years before time 2, the score was at its highest, 1.0. The other subject with fluent aphasia, BS, seems to have no inflectional errors. The figures for DrO probably say more about the methodology than about recovery but do demonstrate that, even on a comparatively simple index, some fluent aphasic speakers will not match normal controls in terms of realising correct inflection, as we assume non-aphasic speakers would have an index of 1.0. Also, very importantly, performance may fluctuate not only between patients but also over time for a single patient.

The second index used in that study which is of interest at this point is an elaboration index, that is, 'average number of open-class words used to elaborate each noun and verb phrase' beyond a noun or a verb. Both subjects with fluent aphasia, BS and DrO, had low scores on this index. The authors state that both subjects with fluent aphasia use 'less well-formed sentences than the controls' and use less 'structural elaboration' (p. 194). No further details are given. Both of the fluent aphasic speakers became better at producing well-formed sentences, an improvement which the authors suggest results from improved lexical accessing (p. 203). This can only be a tentative conclusion, however, as there are problems with the methodology; for example, sample size is not held constant. Despite the problems with this paper, it does serve to illustrate that deficits that at one time were considered to be diagnostic of agrammatism are also found in speakers with fluent aphasia.

We have seen how Butterworth and Howard reject the notion that inflectional errors arise from a grammatical deficit. In fact, they reject the idea that the presence of paragrammatism implicates the grammar at all. The fact that inflection errors appear in fluent aphasia, although not with the same frequency as they do in agrammatism, now seems to be pretty well agreed (Goodglass 1993, Davis 2000), although to date there is no satisfactory account of why this should be so. Studies in languages other than English have also produced evidence that grammar is not always well preserved in fluent aphasia and we will continue to look at some of these errors starting with a study in Finnish.

Niemi (1990:391) examined 'deviations in paragrammatic sentences' that were due to 'non-lexical grammatical components'. Using a large sample of Finnish aphasic speech collected from two speakers, he looked at a number of structural variables. Under what he considered to be *syntax*, he looked at the use of complex NPs, the order of subject and the tensed verb and surface case marking. He also examined text features and pragmatic structure, but we will just examine the features that he considered to be syntactic. He found that the speakers with fluent aphasia produced fewer complex subjects than the non-aphasic speakers. All the speakers were unlikely to produce subjects with embedded clauses, but those with fluent aphasia did so statistically less frequently than the non-fluent speakers. The aphasic speakers were also more likely to use the canonical word order, that is, with subject initial rather than subject final. Cleft and dislocated sentences that were found to be infrequent in non-aphasic speakers were, as might by now be expected, even less frequent in fluent aphasic speech. Niemi claims that these differences cannot be reconciled with the notion that the structural problems arise from lexical difficulties. He further goes on to demonstrate that word order also differs in that speakers with Wernicke's aphasia are much more likely to use the canonical order. They also tend to use the 'morphologically marked partitive and genitive case' more than non-aphasic speakers. In fact they tend to overuse the oblique, the partitive and the accusative and underuse the nominative (morphologically the simplest form). The final piece of evidence that Niemi presents is that his subjects with fluent aphasia used fewer verb ellipses. Niemi suggests that the need to realise the verb phonetically may be linked with the aphasic speaker's need for the verb in order to realise the associated arguments.

Niemi quite rightly acknowledges that these 'abnormalities' or, rather, reduced rate of using certain structures, word order or case, do not necessarily provide evidence of a linguistic deficit, which he glosses as 'loss of language' (p. 402). But there is something amiss here and, at the very least, he suggests that these differences can be characterised as a processing deficit. These findings, while new for Finnish are not entirely new. Gleason, Goodglass, Obler, Green, Hyde and Weintraub (1980) found that their subjects with Wernicke's aphasia used fewer embeddings and relative clauses than their non-aphasic controls. A more recent study by Edwards and Bastiaanse (1998), comparing Dutch and English speakers with fluent aphasia, found that their English fluent aphasic speakers used fewer subordinate clauses than their controls, although this finding was not significant for the Dutch subjects.

The Edwards and Bastiaanse study reports on investigations into lexical as well as grammatical features of fluent aphasic speech. The grammatical feature examined was the ability to produce subordinate clauses and whether this was related to lexical accessing difficulties. They found that the English-speaking aphasics produced subordination less frequently than the non-aphasic speakers. Butterworth and Howard had observed that their fluent aphasics could produce complex sentences but had made no further analysis and had not looked at frequency. Of the ten English aphasic subjects, all but one produced fewer subordinate clauses than the normal controls. However, a different picture was found for the Dutch aphasic speakers. All but one of these speakers produced subordinate clauses as often as the controls, although the number of subordinate clauses used by the Dutch speakers was, unaccountably, considerably lower than the number used by the English speakers. The findings of Edwards and Bastiaanse were in line with those of Gleason, Goodglass, Obler, Green, Hyde and Weintraub (1980) who also found a reduction in complex sentences in their fluent aphasic data.

Could the well-attested lexical problems experienced by these speakers account for the low number of subordinate clauses in the English aphasic data? The authors argued that, if it were the case, then one would expect to find that the ability to use main clauses would also be affected. If a lexical retrieval problem is thought to cause less subordination, then the proportion of main clauses produced should also be affected. In fact this was the case for some, but not all, subjects. Most of the English and all of the Dutch aphasic speakers, produced a similar proportion of main clauses as the normal speakers and, importantly, five of the English aphasic speakers, produced a normal proportion of main clauses but a small proportion of subordinate clauses compared with control speakers. So, having found that some fluent aphasic speakers can produce main clauses but have difficulty with subordinate clauses, is there any clear relationship between these speakers' difficulties with complex sentences and lexical access? One might guess that, for example, a weakness in lexical accessing might have graver consequences when the grammatical demands are greater. If this were true, then those subjects who show difficulties with complex sentences should also demonstrate difficulties with lexical accessing. In fact, this was not seen to be the case, at least on the measures used in this study. It was found that there was no clear association between noun production and clause production. A low number of noun tokens did not predict a low number of either main or subordinate clauses. Even more surprisingly, a low number of verb tokens was not associated with a low proportion of subordinate clauses. In short, the authors conclude that a lexical explanation is insufficient to account for their findings. They noted that fluent aphasic subjects have been found to be poor on some grammatical processing tasks and they query whether the reduced proportion of subordinate clauses might reflect slow grammatical processing.

Verb arguments

There are several features of fluent aphasic speech that are associated with incomplete realisation of obligatory verb arguments in speech. Firstly, failure to complete sentences may lead to failure to supply all the obligatory verb arguments if the NP that is not realised is an obligatory argument. Secondly, lack of all obligatory verb arguments may arise if the non-target verb is retrieved. For example, a fluent aphasic speaker when describing a picture of the Dinner Party, said

(28)   *and she's (er er) putting on a saucepan and stirring it*

The phrasal verb *putting on* cannot be used with *saucepan*. He could have said *she is putting on the tea* or *she is putting the saucepan on the cooker*. Thirdly, the lexical item produced in the verb slot may be a NP instead of a verb, or a NP may be inflected to produce a pseudo-verb. For example, data collected by Clare McCann and Kate Tucker in our aphasia laboratory include the following example:

(29)   *he's choclating* (target: *choosing*)

Whereas these errors may arise because of verb retrieval difficulties, the effect spreads to the verb arguments. If these speakers have incomplete representation of all verb arguments, as had been suggested and will be further discussed in chapter 6, then they will be poor at monitoring these errors. This is certainly the case for many of these speakers who make few, if any, attempts to correct their ill-formed sentences. The intonation used by the speaker often suggests that the speaker is content with the incomplete sentence.

Summary

What we are seeing here, then, from evidence collected from a number of studies, is a range of deficits that fluent aphasic speakers exhibit, all of which can be regarded as paragrammatism. Verb inflection is compromised, sentences are often ill-formed and there is a reduction in the frequency of subordinate clauses. The use of incorrect verb arguments or omission of obligatory arguments are found in this condition. In Finnish there is a reduction in the use of complex NPs in subject position, and word order tends to be canonical. All these observations suggest that the grammar is not functioning well in fluent aphasia. Most of these observations have been taken from spontaneous speech data and are open to interpretation, as we have seen. Later in the monograph we will examine some empirical data where experiments have been set up to allow us to observe details of language processing. We will see how these data add further to the picture of the involvement of the grammar in fluent aphasia.

This chapter concludes with a transcript of a fluent aphasic speaker trying to explain her problems with speaking.

> *I was paralysed (er) right side and I could not cannot talk at all except the (X) and and (er) my par par paralysed arm, leg was . . . it's all right after a week . . . my face was all right after a month but my sneep was very bad and I went to speak therapy and (XX) now . . . go speak therapy but before I could not talk at all . . . I wrote (er) on paper but I cannot understand grammar and it's very hard. For example, I went I want to go to Tesco's. I said . . . I wrote on the note what . . . car . . . some can understand . . . some cannot (er) (X) and them I was very frustrated. Now I can talk better.*

3 *Assessment and fluent aphasia*

Introduction to some aphasia assessments

The presence of aphasia is suspected when there is a sudden loss of language ability usually accompanied by other neuropathological signs. Aphasia may be manifested by problems with the production of words and sentences while comprehension remains relatively intact. People presenting with aphasia who are taken into medical care in the UK will have an aphasia assessment. This will involve a clinician administering various tests but the nature of the tests used will depend on the discipline of the clinician conducting the assessment. Physicians and other medical personnel may run through a few simple tasks such as asking patients to give their name and address, to name a few common objects, a watch, a pen, a glass of water and to point to various objects in the room. This type of exercise contributes to the medical diagnosis but cannot really be thought of as an aphasia assessment. Aphasia assessments, while varying in content, detail and focus, all aim to provide information about the type of disorder rather than the presence of aphasia. If the patient enters into a rehabilitation programme, then an assessment may be given to establish baselines before clinical intervention and to check change in language performance over time, in order to inform the planning of therapy.

Inexperienced speech and language therapists and those with insufficient time to allow them to deal adequately with aphasia may use short screening tests, which identify the presence of aphasia and give some scores in very general terms such as 'expression' and 'comprehension'. Such screening offers little information about the nature of the language disorder and is so basic that mild aphasia may go undetected. Assessments are rarely given to establish the presence of aphasia if the clinician is knowledgeable about aphasia. A short conversation is usually sufficient for the experienced clinician to confirm that aphasia is present and the same short, initial informal conversation may also be used to check certain features of connected speech. A more detailed look at the use of connected speech as a means of assessing aphasia will be given in chapter 4.

Here, in this chapter, we will consider some published aphasia assessments that comprise a number of tasks that are used to examine the disorder and to yield information about the nature of the language disorder.

Whereas the presence of aphasia is usually obvious, testing is occasionally necessary to differentiate between early dementia and fluent aphasia. However, part of the diagnosis of dementia arises from observation of deviant behaviour. Language may be disordered in dementia but is accompanied by concomitant changes in non-linguistic behaviour, such as reduction in memory capacity and in inhibition, paranoia and changes in social skills. In contrast, in aphasia, non-linguistic behaviour remains much as it was before the incident that caused the aphasia. Of course, if the brain damage that caused the stroke also caused other deficits, such as paralysis or visual problems, then these deficits would limit the range of behaviours available to the person with aphasia. The person may have reduced mobility with serious social consequences. Visual problems may restrict activities and there may be some changes in memory capacity. As a result of these changes, the person may become dependent, to a greater or lesser degree, on others and have to come to terms with a major change in his or her role within the family, work and social environments. That person, under-standably, may also experience various levels of depression, although human nature is remarkably resilient and depression not inevitable by any means. But, not withstanding these physical and social changes and the change in language behaviour, the person with aphasia remains much the same person as before the incident, in that non-verbal behaviour remains within normal bounds and is not deviant. There is a different picture when the person has dementia, as then behaviour becomes increasingly bizarre. So, although the person with dementia may have language problems, especially word-finding difficulties that resemble fluent aphasia, a person with dementia can usually be distinguished from one with aphasia. That being the case, a differential diagnosis is usually straight-forward.

That is not to say that errors in diagnosis never happen. They do, especially if the person with fluent aphasia has a history of psychiatric illness and the person responsible for the initial diagnosis is a physician with limited experience of language disorders. The following case illustrates this. The person concerned had a history of depression and anxiety, conditions for which medication had been prescribed and were thus recorded in the medical notes. This person, a recently retired highly educated man, was also in a very volatile marriage. When the stroke occurred, the person, realising that something was amiss, admitted himself to a local Accident and Emergency Department. He was in a very stressed state and was incoherent. The medical notes were consulted and the doctor on duty thought the patient was in an extreme state of anxiety bordering on psychosis and admitted the man to a psychiatric ward. Realising what was happening, the man became even more distressed and agitated and so the situation escalated. It took a few days for the medical personnel to realise their mistake, whereas, had there been an attempt to test his language abilities or to explore whether an aphasia was present, then, provided that the examiner had the adequate expertise, the correct diagnosis would have been arrived at on admission. However, the extreme agitation and anxiety exhibited by the patient caused the doctors to justify their decision. After all, the patient did respond favourably to the medication given. That is, the anxiety abated. The aphasia, however, remained as florid and as severe as at the time of admission. Eventually, after considerable delay, the patient was referred to speech and language therapy. Fortunately, such cases are rare.

So occasionally a test to reveal the presence of aphasia can be useful, especially for nursing and medical staff, but assessment of aphasia is much more commonly performed, not to establish the existence of aphasia, but to reveal details of the aphasia. Those details will include some kind of estimation of the severity of the language impairment in production and understanding. Deficits vary in type and severity within the domains of the sound system, the lexicon and the grammar. Although there is a fair amount of variation across subjects, patterns of deficits occur. The knowledge that patterns occur in aphasia influences the structure of all assessments, but researchers have differing views as to what these patterns are and assessments reflect this range of views. We will start with a general overview of tests and the motivation behind their development. We will then consider three assessments that are widely used in clinical practice and research. A brief overview of two more recently published assessments that illustrate the changes that have taken place in the mode of assessment and the focus of assessment will follow. Finally, we will consider in some detail a battery of tests that has been developed to investigate the understanding and production of verbs and sentences in aphasia, which yields a different quality of information.

Assessing aphasia in a clinical context

Two tests frequently used are the Boston Diagnostic Aphasia Examination (BDAE; Goodglass and Kaplan 1972, 1983, Goodglass, Kaplan and Barresi 2001) and the Western Aphasia Battery (WAB; Kertesz 1982). Both of these tests use the traditional notion of syndrome and the view that the patterns of language deficit associated with aphasic syndromes (a) are indicative of the loci of the cerebral lesion and (b) can be bundled into syndromes. When the tests were first published, technology did not offer the range of neurological investigations that are now available, and what was available was not part of normal clinical practice. Thus a test that could give some information about lesion site was considered to be clinically important. During the last twenty years, however, the range of available investigations has multiplied and now information about lesion site is often given routinely following a neurological examination and, as a result, the diagnosis of lesion site is not of primary interest in the aphasia assessment. However, as the notion of syndrome is so closely linked with lesion site and, as the notion of syndrome persists, especially within the research literature, a test that can select patients or experimental subjects by diagnostic type is still considered to be useful. Indeed, several academic journals insist that authors include diagnostic information in their subject description.

The new version of the BDAE (Goodglass, Kaplan and Barresi 2001) includes a shortened version of the original test and a range of other sub-tests for extended investigations. The aims of the test remain the same as for the two previous versions: to diagnose the presence and types of aphasia and to assess and measure performance on a range of language tasks in order to guide therapy. The publication of this new version of the BDAE and the continued use of the WAB testify to clinicians' use of diagnostic categories. The use of the syndromic framework is widespread in the international research community and acts as a common reference point for those conducting research. The alternative, as Grodzinsky (1991) and others claim, is to consider each and every case as unique. Now, whereas individual variability is not disputed, if we are to look for explanations of the language deficits then we need to look for commonalities. That is what the syndromic framework provides. There is a whole raft of research that starts from the premise that aphasia symptoms vary across subjects, but it can be useful to think of aphasia as a collection of syndromes. Each syndrome represents a collection of symptoms that co-occur more frequently than by chance. The symptoms include deficits within different domains of language, deficits of sentence construction, of verb inflection and of lexical retrieval. As we have seen, deficits of grammar and lexis are thought to dissociate in Broca's and Wernicke's aphasia. Thus investigations of aphasia within these syndrome groups gives, it is argued, not only diagnostic information but also insight into the separate domains of language.

Work driven by hypotheses such as the neuro-anatomical representation of specific components of the grammar needs to establish distinct experimental groups. In order to do this, subjects need to be tested by a procedure that is

generally accepted within the research community or, as is more likely in aphasiology, at least accepted within their corner of the research field. Thus these
assessment protocols are frequently used in order to group subjects on the basis
of these syndromes for research purposes. Examples of such work would be
an investigation into verb deficits in non-fluent and fluent aphasic speakers
(Zingeser and Berndt 1990), or an examination of how argument structure
affects verb accessing in non-fluent aphasic subjects versus fluent aphasic subjects (Shapiro, Gordon, Hack and Killackey 1993).

Clinical research also utilises single case-study designs and group designs
to explore the nature of aphasia and the effect of aphasia therapy. Most of
the reported therapy research is with single subjects or small group studies
(most of these being with agrammatic patients rather than patients with fluent
aphasia). The single-subject design is the preferred research methodology for
some researchers while others argue that such designs are inappropriate. If
a treatment regime is seen to be effective, then it is of limited interest to the
practising clinician unless the information can be applied to other patients. If the
effective therapy is the result of treating one patient, and that patient is described
only in terms of his or her individual profile of deficits, then the possibility of
using this treatment effectively with other patients depends on the rare chance of
finding another patient whose deficits match exactly. However, if the patient is
described as having a type of aphasia, say agrammatism, or Wernicke's aphasia,
then similar patients can be found and the treatment regime applied to a type
or group of patients.

The variety of testing materials

There is a plethora of materials available for the assessment of aphasia. In the
early days these were modelled on psychometric assessments, starting with the
Language Modality Test for Aphasia (Wepman and Jones 1961). For years, tests
were developed using this model, testing language through the four 'modalities'
of speaking, listening, reading and writing, and consisting of a series of tasks
involving listening and responding to language, elicited speech, and written
and reading tasks. Test protocols involved responding to various commands,
naming pictured or real objects, repeating words, reciting numbers, and days of
the week and so on. Both the BDAE and the WAB have followed this format, as
has the Aachen Aphasia Test (Huber, Poeck, Weniger and Willmes 1983). The
Aachen Aphasia Test was originally produced in German but has subsequently
been adapted for a number of European languages. Most recently, it has been
adapted for use with English-speaking aphasic patients (Miller, Willmes and

De Bleser 2000). The Aachen still follows the format of the BDAE and WAB although it claims to reflect 'patterns of linguistic structure'. Rather confusingly, it also claims to investigate: (1) *levels* of language (phonology, semantics and syntax); (2) *units* of language (described as phonemes, morphemes and syntactic structures); and (3) the *rules* applied to the combination of these units.

There are some other tests that have been developed in the last twenty years or so that reflect the growth in knowledge about aphasic and non-aphasic language. Many of these tests have abandoned any attempt to assess language in all four modalities through a collection of spoken and written tasks, as do the BDAE, the WAB and the Aachen, but seek to expose details of one or more deficits associated with aphasia. Tests have been devised that are less general, focusing on, say, the ability to assess a patient's ability to produce nouns via a picture-naming task, for example the Boston Naming Test (Goodglass, Kaplan and Weintraub 1983). Most tests now take account of at least some psycholinguistic features of language, such as word frequency when testing single-word comprehension and production, and some take account of short-term memory and latency of response. However, despite developments in linguistic theories, there has been little attempt to explore grammar to any great extent or to develop tests motivated by any linguistic theory.

In addition to the tests specifically designed for aphasia assessment, tests that have not been specifically designed for aphasia assessment are also used. Some of these tests have the added advantage that they have been standardised on a normal population whereas not all aphasia assessments have been. Since it is assumed that non-aphasic subjects will score at or near 100 per cent on all parts of the test, the assessments do not necessarily include a range of scores for non-aphasic controls. Unfortunately, the control groups tend to be small. During standardisation of the English Aachen Aphasia Test, the test was given to three control groups: a healthy group of 24 subjects; a group of 41 hospitalised patients with no language problems; and a group of 28 speakers with neurological illnesses but no language problems. Results from all these non-aphasic speakers were compared with the results obtained from 93 subjects with aphasia. The test discriminated between the two groups (aphasic and non-aphasic), with the normal controls making hardly any errors on any of the sub-tests (Miller, Willmes and De Bleser 2000:701). In the 1982 standardisation of the Boston Diagnostic Aphasia Examination, the control group was much larger: 147 neurologically normal males between the ages of 25 and 85 years old. The mean for most sub-tests was 'within a fraction of the maximum score' although some individuals fell below by five or six points. The authors therefore give cut-off points for each sub-test (Goodglass and Kaplan 1983:28).

Some tests used with the aphasic population have been standardised with children. For example the Test for the Reception of Grammar (TROG; Bishop 1982) tests sentence comprehension, incorporating grammatical contrasts such as plurals, locative pronouns, relative clauses and so on and is sometimes used to test understanding of spoken sentences when difficulties in parsing syntax is suspected. Results may then be used to motivate therapy with non-fluent aphasic people but to date no consistent pattern of deficits has been revealed by this test. British Picture Vocabulary Scales (Dunn, Dunn, Wetton and Burley 1997) that has scores for children up to the age of 15;08 may be used to supplement naming tests designed for aphasia assessment, for, unlike many aphasia tests, it is not restricted to nouns and therefore gives a broader picture.

Aphasia therapists in the UK are all speech and language therapists, working within limited resources and with limited opportunities to experiment with a wide range of assessments. They tend to work with tests they are familiar with and that are available. Often the popularity of an assessment is dependent on the ease with which it can be administered and the amount of publicity surrounding the launch of the test rather than on the detail of information revealed about the language disorder. Of course, the therapist is looking for a test that yields useful information about the disorder but is often unwilling or unable to devote the necessary time and effort to explore the nature of what is a very complicated language disorder. It is not unusual, at least in the UK, to find people with aphasia who have undergone no standard assessment several months post-onset. This situation is likely to change, however, to meet the needs of clinical audit.

Tests vary in content, structure, detail and underlying philosophies. The simplest tests aim to reveal the presence of aphasia. There are then a bunch of tests that aim to diagnose the type of aphasia. At the simplest level, diagnosis may be limited to deciding whether comprehension or production of language is the more impaired, while tests developed in the 1980s seek to diagnose a patient in terms of one of the classical aphasia syndromes. We will now review some of the most frequently used assessments, focusing on their ability to reveal meaningful details about fluent aphasia. As an example, we will discuss results obtained, on a range of tests and over a period of time, for MG, our subject with fluent aphasia. Following this, a new test that investigates the understanding and production of verbs and sentences in aphasia will be introduced and data collected from people with fluent aphasia will be examined. We will see how fluent aphasic speakers cope with tasks involving the production of verbs and sentences and how their abilities differ, if at all, from speakers with non-fluent aphasia.

The Boston Diagnostic Aphasia Examination (BDAE)

Probably the most influential assessment to emerge in the latter half of the twentieth century was the Boston Diagnostic Aphasia Examination (Goodglass and Kaplan 1972, 1983) and it is therefore worth spending some time considering this test. There has been a recent revision (Goodglass, Kaplan and Barresi 2001) which contains a clinic-friendly short-form of the test and some further updated tests to use. These reflect some of the psycholinguistic research conducted in the last twenty years or so. In most respects, the new BDAE is essentially the same test as the earlier versions of the BDAE. As the title suggests, the purpose of this assessment is diagnostic, aiming not merely to diagnose the presence of aphasia but also to establish the type of aphasia present. The types of aphasia recognised by Goodglass and colleagues are neoclassic in that they echo the types of aphasia identified by aphasiologists, in the main neurologists working and publishing at the end of the nineteenth century and at the beginning of the twentieth century. It is the wide use of this assessment for clinical and research purposes that has established the notion of the division of aphasia into non-fluent and fluent types, each of which is then further subdivided into one of the classical aphasic types, also known as syndromes.

Fluency as a diagnostic feature

Fluency as a diagnostic feature is a notion that has been around a long time. In the sixties, Geschwind and Howes noted that the spontaneous output of aphasic speakers fell into two distinct categories, fluent and non-fluent (Howes 1964, Howes and Geschwind 1964, Geschwind 1966). This distinction was taken up by other researchers, such as Benson (1967), who found a correlation between these two broad types of aphasia and site of lesion. Goodglass (Geschwind's student) and Kaplan used this dichotomy in the development of their assessment and borrowed the dimensions of phrase length, used earlier by Benson. As Poeck (1989:24) points out, this distinction was rapidly accepted in the scientific community even though the distinction has never been based on a fixed set of criteria. In the Assessment of Aphasia, Goodglass and Kaplan (1983:6) give the following guide on how to recognise fluent aphasic speech:

> Fluency is best rated in terms of the longest occasional uninterrupted strings
> of words that are produced.

They claim that 'fluency is best judged from speech production during an extended conversation and free narrative'.

Albert, Goodglass, Helm, Rubens and Alexander (1981:4) state that there are three important distinctions to be made for the purpose of gross clinical diagnosis. One of these is the distinction between fluent and non-fluent aphasia. (The other two being the presence or absence of a repetition deficit and the third being the distinction between oral and written language disorders.) They describe fluent speech as:

> Speech that is produced at a normal rate, with normal speech rhythm and melody, good articulation and normal or hyper-normal phrase length.

Albert et al. elaborated on the descriptions given by Goodglass and Kaplan and produced a more detailed account of how fluency can be recognised. We will use their definitions of the defining features of fluency that appear in the BDAE as they give slightly more information than Goodglass and Kaplan. The assessment of fluency takes into account a number of features. The examiner is asked to assess what is called the 'melodic line', which is based on 'the normal intonation pattern of a sentence' (Albert et al. 1981:26), that is, whether or not the speaker maintains intonation patterns. 'Phrase length' is another defining feature, which, again according to Albert et al., 'does not refer to grammatical phrases but merely to the number of words uttered between pauses'. The third defining feature of fluent aphasia according to the BDAE is 'articulatory agility', defined as speech that sounds 'normally agile' in contrast to the effortful speech of the non-fluent aphasic speaker. There are obvious problems with these definitions, not only in their lack of clarity but also in the lack of any point of contact with what is known about language, especially in the present context. Yet, despite their lack of precision and of linguistic sophistication, they still act as rather gross descriptive terms of fluent aphasia. It is still recognised that fluent aphasic speech does have normal intonation, tends to have sentence structure preserved, at least compared with non-fluent aphasia, and, although phonemic paraphasic errors may be present, this disorder is not associated with effortful or dyspraxic articulation. The final feature highlighted as a characteristic of fluent aphasia, 'a variety of grammatical forms', is also, in very general terms and especially if taken in contrast to non-fluent aphasia, fairly easily recognised. However, for this feature, the authors provide a definition that is not applicable and is slightly at odds with the description given by Goodglass and Kaplan (1983). Albert et al. state that this fluent aphasic speech is characterised by a 'variety of syntactic forms with no tendency to omit grammatical function words or inflectional forms (1981:30). Goodglass and Kaplan's (1983:80) description differs slightly in that they add that 'the grammar of (fluent aphasic speakers) is often incorrect' although described as 'paragrammatic' rather than 'agrammatic'. We have seen in earlier chapters that there is mounting evidence that fluent aphasic speakers do make grammatical errors and that there have been some endeavours to examine these errors.

The two categories of fluent and non-fluent have been termed superstructures, each of which embrace several of the traditional aphasic syndromes (Poeck 1989), and so the actual characteristics of these two broad types of aphasia can vary considerably. However, as a broad rule of thumb, the fluent aphasic speaker will be more proficient at constructing sentences than the non-fluent aphasic speaker, and this dimension holds for all four types of fluent aphasia (anomia, conduction aphasia, Wernicke's aphasia and transcortical sensory aphasia). What is surprising about the Boston Diagnostic Aphasia Examination is that there is no objective test for fluency/non-fluency. The features discussed above are components of a profile that the examiner compiles based on listening to a sample of spontaneous speech collected via a picture-description task, but there are no guidelines for objective scoring of this task. The decision whether the patient is fluent or non-fluent is based on a rating scale profile where the examiner must score the aphasic speaker on seven features: melodic line, phrase length, grammatical form, paraphasia in running speech, repetition, word finding and auditory comprehension. Only the last three items are based on scores obtained in the test battery, the other four from observation of performance and, in particular, from the picture-description task. The sub-tests of this battery give some objective quantification of various language tasks. They cover different types of naming tasks, repetition of single words and sentences and reading. The aim of the test is to assess the 'components of language' using the four modalities of speaking, listening, writing and reading as 'windows' through which language capacity can be viewed. This, the authors say, contrasts with Wepman's aim to test the functioning of each modality (Goodglass and Kaplan 1983:3).

Western Aphasia Battery

Kertesz (1982) produced a very similar assessment battery, the Western Aphasia Battery. He claims that in his battery, fluency is rated according to a set of criteria based on replies to a set of questions and a picture description. Each patient is assigned a fluency score ranging from 0 to 10. Scores depend on whether 'short meaningless utterances' are uttered (in which case a zero score is awarded), or the utterances are 'sentences of normal length and complexity, without perceptible word-finding difficulty' (in which case the maximum score of 10 is gained). Each level contains a hotchpotch of features such as 'hesitancy over parts of speech, auxiliary verbs or word endings', jargon, 'more complete propositional phrases' and so on. Given this mixture of items that describe production characteristics that include features of speed, features of lexical access, syntactic morphological features and meaning, it is hard to take the notion of 'fluency' seriously. Yet it persists as a useful descriptive term both in clinical practice and in research. It serves as a shorthand notion and captures the salient feature of two aphasic types that at least sound very different from each other and that usually arise from different lesion sites.

Classification

Perhaps a more urgent concern for those wishing to use syndromic classifications is the low number of cases that can be accurately classified in these schemes. We have already mentioned in chapter 1 that Goodglass and his colleagues acknowledged that not all patients could be classified by the Boston schemes and how de Bleser and her colleagues found a poor fit even when selecting 'typical' cases. Crary and associates (1992) compared the BDAE with the WAB and found that only 38 per cent of those classified on the Boston corresponded to the syndromes of the WAB and, further, only 30 per cent of those classified on the WAB corresponded with those classified by the Boston. It is therefore important to remember that findings from research that have used the classical syndromes may be generalisable only to a small proportion of the clinical population.

The assessments that use these terms, while orientating the examiner to salient features of aphasia and giving some information about the aphasic speaker's ability to do certain tasks, offer little ready information on the nature of the language disorder. The results leave the investigator with a fair amount of work to do in order to discover any details about the lexical or grammatical deficits or anything about possible underlying processes. It is not surprising, then, given the limitations of these tests and the growth in knowledge about language, that new assessments continue to be produced despite the longevity of the tests first designed over thirty years ago. Some new tests tend to be variations of the Boston although the construction may reflect more sophisticated psychometrics. We will look at some of these more recent tests below, but first let us examine an example of BDAE profile. The Boston profile was used with this patient as it is part of the common currency of aphasia therapists in the UK and allows comparisons across research data and clinical data. The test covers the four modalities of spoken and written language input and output, tests language in terms of single words and connected speech, and the results of these tests suggest areas for further detailed investigations. Descriptions of the Cookie Theft picture (part of the BDAE) abound in the literature, allowing direct comparisons to be made between speech samples collected from a variety of sources. The whole of the test can be completed in a reasonable time so that profiles can be collected for a series of patients. Testing on the BDAE is usually stage one of the assessment process. Further probing in specific areas, for example, word retrieval, would employ further tools, perhaps sub-tests from PALPA. This can be considered as stage two of the assessment process, as PALPA has been designed for detailed, specific investigation, and not for obtaining an overall profile.

An example of a BDAE profile

The subject, MG, has been examined by the BDAE on several occasions. The first record of the test was at three months post-onset of his aphasia and since then he has been examined at irregular intervals over a number of years. As has been explained above, the BDAE produces a number of test results and it is partly on the basis of these results and partly on the clinician's judgement that a profile and a severity score are gained.

So how was MG diagnosed as having Wernicke's aphasia? A CT scan showed that there had been an infarct in the left middle cerebral artery distribution that involved cortical and sub-cortical white matter over an extensive area especially in the left temporal and adjacent parietal lobe. The profile of test scores and the speech characteristics of MG in the early stages post-onset of aphasia (seven months after the stroke) was typical of this type of lesion and best fitted the profile given by Goodglass and Kaplan for a Wernicke's aphasic. His 'phrase length' was at five words, slightly below their lower limit and grammatical form was not scored, maybe because the clinician, not surprisingly, found this difficult to score. His repetition ability and auditory comprehension, scores transferred from the test part of the assessment, were also within the Wernicke's profile, as was the number of paraphasic errors noted in the naming tasks. This result matched the therapist's clinical judgement, that he was described as a patient with fluent aphasia typical of Wernicke's aphasia, and provided a base line whereby language change over the coming years could be measured. It did not, however, tell the therapist much about the nature of the errors that were made in his speech or about the nature of the difficulties he had with understanding the language of others around him.

At ten months post-onset the profile for MG shows the following: he was using phrases of five words; grammatical form was found to be just below

Table 3.1 *MG's scores expressed as percentiles for naming and comprehension tasks on the Boston Diagnostic Aphasia Examination*

Date of testing	Naming		Animal names	Word disc.	Body parts	Comprehension	
	Responsive	Confrontational				Commands	Complex
7/1990	50	15	—	50+	60	20	40
10/1990	60+	45	—	60	45	70	50
8/1992	40+	65	90	60	80	60	50
4/1993	40+	85	90	50	80	30	50
10/1994	80+	80	90	60+	—	65	60
11/1996	65	75	90+	40	50	65	60

the normal range; there were paraphasic errors in every utterance; repetition for single words was intact but for phrases and sentences it was poor; and the average score on the comprehension tests was 60 per cent.

A further set of scores is available for MG at three years post-onset of the aphasia and there were some notable improvements in some of his scores. His 'phrase length' was roughly the same as would be expected. Typically, for Wernicke's aphasia, it was near normal although the number of errors in his production resulted in many of the utterances being intelligible. Paraphasic errors were reduced from 'present in every utterance' to 'once per minute of conversation' and his naming ability had increased on the tests. However, his 'word-finding' score based on spontaneous speech was judged to be the same, and the mean percentile of four comprehension sub-tests was still hovering around the 50th percentile. Despite the fact that he had become a better communicator, he still presented with aphasia and that, according to the Boston profile, was still Wernicke's aphasia.

The above scores are taken from the Sub-test Summary Profile of the BDAE and need to be read with caution. All scores are converted to percentiles on this summary profile, which aids comparison across tests with varying numbers of items. The percentiles are given in tens and therefore the resulting profile scores gloss any small progress made between testing. Thus the scores given above record an improvement in MG's ability to name pictures (the confrontational naming section), to produce a list of animal names and to follow commands, but the fine details are lost. Furthermore the test scores do not indicate changes in his spontaneous speech or his understanding of day-to-day communication. Information gained provides some limited data that can act as a base-line against which future changes can be compared. However, it gives no details about the nature of the language deficit.

The scores do show that the aphasia diminished over a four-year period, although there are some anomalies. First we see that, according to these scores, performance on obeying commands after the initial improvement is somewhat erratic. This could reflect poor inter-tester reliability (although we would hope that our testers are consistent and reliable), or it could reflect fluctuations in the subject's concentration. We have to assume that the underlying language processes are intact otherwise good performance could not pre-date poor. Further, as there is only one section where a drop in performance occurs, we assume it is neither a general decrease in language abilities nor unreliable testing. Finally, we note that the last profile compiled six years post-onset of the aphasia shows a decrease in two of the naming scores and two of the comprehension scores. The two comprehension scores that do not decrease reflect more accurately his comprehension of everyday speech while the single-word comprehension has decreased. There is no ready explanation for these variations although they may reflect some regression of performance linked to absence of treatment. This pattern is the reverse of that discussed by Inglis (2003) in a study that contrasts improvement in scores without overt training. There are very few data on long-term language performance in aphasia despite the relatively long life expectancy of many people with aphasia.

A daughter of the BDAE: the Aachen Aphasia Test

The Aachen Aphasia Test (Huber, Poeck, Weniger and Willmes 1983, Huber, Poeck and Willmes 1984) and the recent English version of the test (Miller, Willmes and De Bleser 2000) have a similar structure to the BDAE and the WAB. Like these two tests, the Aachen test is a diagnostic test providing exemplars of various aphasic syndromes against which a patient's profile can be compared. And, like the BDAE and the WAB, it tests language functioning in the modalities of speech and written language. It also assesses repetition abilities. It explicitly sets out to investigate three aspects of language: different domains of language, units within these domains and rules governing the combination of the units. The authors describe this as 'the levels (phonology, semantics, syntax)', 'units of language (phonemes, morphemes and syntactic structures)' and 'the regularities, or rules that apply . . . for the combination and differentiation of these units' (Miller, Willmes and de Bleser 2000:680). There are six parts to the test: a spontaneous speech sample; a version of the Token Test; a test of repetition; written language; naming; and comprehension.

Scoring of the spontaneous speech is rated on a six-point scale that includes rating of phonological, semantic and syntactic structure, articulation and prosody and, rather strangely, formulaic language. In the naming section, subjects are required to name pictured objects, colours, pictured compound nouns and pictured sentences. The ten sentences elicited vary in length, some having more complex NPs than others, for example *father and son are playing cowboys and Indians* compared with *the man is begging*, but all have the same SVO structure. The final sentence is more complex as it involves verb ellipsis and two coordinated clauses, *the man is lying on the couch, smoking a pipe and reading a newspaper.*

While there has been a lot of attention paid to the trialling of the English version of the test, and certain psychometric factors have been taken into account, noticeably word frequency and sentence length, there seems to be little evidence that the results of this test will do any more than assign patients to aphasia syndromes much as the tests developed thirty years or so ago. Confusingly (for students, at least), the syndromes used in the Aachen differ from those used in the BDAE although there is some overlap. Certainly, the examiner will be able to collect examples of phonological and syntactic errors, but this test will not give any readily available information about a speaker's phonological or syntactic skills. Nor will it give any insights into underlying processes that are faulty. Indeed, the authors state that assignment of subjects to an aphasia category 'rests on surface language performance' and that the test 'makes no assumptions about models of language functioning underlying behaviour'. The aim is, they claim, to 'furnish only a linguistic description of an individual's performance' (p. 685). Given these aims, it is then important to ascertain whether the test (a) categorizes correctly and (b) yields enough data for the application of models.

How might we expect a typical fluent aphasic speaker to perform on this test and what insights can it provide? Our fluent aphasic subject, MG, achieved the following profile seven years post-trauma.

Repetition: MG scored between 80 and 97 per cent for repeating sounds and single words but only 30 per cent for repeating sentences, scores compatible with those achieved on the Boston.

Naming: His naming of objects and colours produced scores between 67 per cent and 87 per cent. There was some difference between his ability to name objects such as *table*, *cigar* and *candle* for which he gained 86 per cent and his ability to name the so-called compound nouns such as *hairdryer* and *windmill* for which he scored 67 per cent.

Sentence production is included in this section. The subject is required to produce a sentence to describe a picture. For this he scored only 30 per cent.

For the target *the teacher is explaining something* he produced *the picture, the girl, the blackboard*.

Auditory comprehension: On these tests he scored 83 per cent for single words and 73 per cent for sentences, rather higher scores than those gained on the BDAE.

On the basis of the profile of his spontaneous speech, he could be classified as having Wernicke's aphasia, but he only partially matched this profile and could equally have been classified *amnestic*, the EAAT term for *anomic* aphasia. Although this is a recently developed test, it does not say much about the nature of the aphasia beyond confirming that this speaker has more problems with producing and understanding sentences than with understanding and producing single words. We do not know *why* sentences are more difficult to understand or if all sentences are equally difficult. There is no way of finding out if syntax is compromised or whether it is a word-finding difficulty that lies at the root of the problem. The next assessment we will look at delves a little deeper into the lexical problems but adds little to our understanding of problems at the sentential level.

The Psycholinguistic Analysis of Language Processing

Not all tests produce a syndromic diagnosis nor do they claim to provide insights into the underlying nature of the language disorder. We have seen how the authors of the English Aachen Aphasia Test have claimed that the test results provide the data to which models of language processing can then be applied. Such tests can be thought of as 'model free'. Few tests produced in the last ten to fifteen years have sought to provide information about the assumed underlying problem with the language processes that exist in aphasia and eschew the notion of syndrome. Although there are a number of inventive protocols reported in the research literature, there are still very few published tests motivated by an explicit model of language processing for the clinician to use. This is surprising considering the dissatisfaction there is with the concept of syndromes and the idea that assessment is about diagnosis of the aphasia type.

A group of researchers working in the UK, abandoning the syndromic approach, started to base much of their work on a model of single-word production, first used in the work on dyslexia (see, e.g., Byng, Kay, Edmonson and Scott 1990). Their work depends on a model of single-word production that has discrete stages that can be independently damaged. Once identified, this is known as 'the level of breakdown'. For example, a problem with word retrieval might arise because the aphasic speaker has problems with meanings of words while another might have problems with the phonological form of words. In the former case, the level of breakdown will be considered to be at the semantic level and in the latter case at the phonological level. The locus of the deficit in the latter case can then be further subdivided, according to errors made, between problems of phonological assembly or problems at the level of the 'phonological buffer', a sort of short-term memory (STM), or phonological loop of the STM. The idea is that several speakers with aphasia may have word-finding difficulties that appear very similar but, when they are given appropriate tests, different causes will emerge. It is important to note that the model has been built to deal only with the production and understanding of nouns and therefore is limited in application.

The Psycholinguistic Analysis of Language Processing in Aphasia (PALPA), test (Kay, Lesser and Coltheart 1994) is built on this premise, that the access to the meaning and phonological form of words can be separately and independently impaired. In this test, nouns are the main focus and there are no tests of verb production or comprehension. It uses a model that seems to consider words as separate and unrelated items, a model that pays no heed to the role of words within sentences or the potential grammatical role of the words tested. The complete battery does include some tests for the production and understanding of closed- versus open-class words and for the understanding of sentences, but its strength lies in providing ways of investigating details of the understanding and production of nouns as single words. Word production is conceived as a process starting from some kind of central semantic module, the nature of which is largely unspecified, leading through various stages of phonological representation to the final stage of muscular activity. It is a fairly simple model of single-word production and, in the authors' own words, under-specified. It offers a limited explanation for the production of some nouns as single words and as a single class but has nothing to say about verbs, determiners, auxiliaries, etc.

Single-word retrieval

Using MG as way of illustrating this test, we can see how the test sets about identifying semantic problems, as we would expect to see in fluent aphasia. MG had problems with word retrieval, making both phonological and lexical paraphasic errors. Investigations using the PALPA confirmed that problems arose at the semantic as well as the phonological level of processing. For example, on a sub-test given three years post-onset that required him to select a word similar in meaning to the target word, he found words with high imageability easier than those with low. He scored 11 out of 15 correct in the high imageability section and 5 in the low imageability test. His errors showed that he selected an unrelated foil more often than a foil that was semantically related to the target, thus suggesting that he wasn't good at accessing the meaning of the words in the test. In a related test administered around the same time, MG was unable to give definitions of words even though he was able to read them. In this test, the regularity of the spelling helped: he scored 9/10 on the section with the 'regularly' spelt words (such as *pale* and *meat*) and only 5/10 on the 'exception' words (such as *bear, roll, heir, suite* and *colonel*). The criteria used in this test for 'regular' and 'exception' are not clear. 'Exception' cannot be the same as 'unique' as *bear* and *roll* are included: compare *wear* and *droll*. The fact that he was better at reading the 'regular' words can be interpreted as MG having access to grapheme-phoneme conversion, thus enabling him to read words that had regular spelling even though he was unable to access, or at least give, the meaning of most of the words. However, phonological representation of words was not intact as MG made errors on tests that probed his ability to judge words that rhymed or shared the same initial phoneme.

Sentence comprehension

The sentence-comprehension sub-tests of the PALPA examine a subject's comprehension of sentences that vary in syntactic structure. The procedure used is a picture selection where the subject is required to select one of four pictures that match a target sentence. Three distractor pictures are used with each target sentence. The distractors are (a) lexical where the same characters are used but a different verb from the target verb is used, (b) reverse roles where the role of agent and theme/patient are reversed and (c) a picture with an event unconnected to the target. All sentences are built around a verb and two NPs and the test includes fourteen different types of sentence structure. The types of sentences used are actives, full passives and a range of other structures probing less transparent factors that contribute to the comprehension of sentences. Some of the active and passive sentences are reversible, that is each of the NPs is a plausible agent or patient. This allows the factor of 'reversibility' to be examined across other sentence structures. The authors have included two types of 'non-reversible comparative sentences'. There are four sentences with a comparative adjective and sentences with a 'to complement' such as *this dog's got more cats to chase*, although they claim that they have 'generally found that 'despite greater length and complexity, these longer comparative sentences do not cause extra difficulty. The difference highlighted here is length of sentence rather than structure and the authors did not point out that the 'longer' comparative sentences also have a more complex syntactic structure (two VPs) and include a gapped NP and movement.

There are other problems with this sub-test. The descriptions of sentence types is muddling and not always accurate. The authors include sentences that they describe as 'gapped after the verb where the gap is a subject' (e.g. *The girl's asking what to eat*). In fact, the gap in this sentence is in the object position, after *to eat*: presumably, the authors are referring to *what*. The authors also refer to sentences with gaps 'after verbs' but, it is claimed, these are gaps 'not as subject' (e.g. *the girl's indicating where to go*). Again this is confusing. Once more the gap is in the object position, after *to go*, and the reader therefore has to conclude that the authors are referring to *where*. Now, *what* and *where* involve different types of movement. *What* is an NP movement and *where* is an adjunct movement. Work by Thompson and her colleagues have demonstrated that this difference is not just a theoretical one but has implications for therapy. However, because this distinction is not made in the PALPA manual, nor many items of each type included, the distinction is likely to be ignored by most people using this test. There are also items that include 'converse relations', that is, sentences that include verbs such as *following* and *buying*. Because only partial syntactic information is given about these sentences, clinicians, unless they are also good syntacticians, are unlikely to discover which syntactic features are problematic.

This sub-test of the PALPA includes thirteen different sentence types although we may disagree with how they describe their sentence types. There are four examples of each sentence type. It is difficult to get a clear pattern of a person's comprehension difficulties using the categories the authors give, where features such as reversibility, 'gapping' and verb types are compounded within single sentences. For example, it is difficult to tell whether 'reversibility' of the NPs used is a factor, as the twenty reversible sentences contain five different sentence structures and the sixteen non-reversible sentences comprise four different sentence types. Four of the non-reversible sentences are comparatives, such as *the girl's got more chickens*, and four sentences include not only comparatives but also subject gaps, such as *the girl's got more horses to feed*. Thus if we want to examine the contribution of lexical knowledge versus syntactic or the effect of gapped NPs, then the examiner needs to search among the sub-tests and is left with a small set of the illustrative sentences and an uneven distribution of items. There are, for example, only four sentences categorised as non-reversible active or passive sentences. However, a further eight sentences are also non-reversible;

Table 3.2 *MG's scores for sentence comprehension from PALPA*

Sentence type	2 years post-onset: number correct		7 years post-onset: number correct	
All actives	9/12	75%	8/12	67%
Non-reversible actives	4/4	100%	4/4	100%
Reversible actives	5/8	62%	4/8	50%
All passives	7/12	58%	8/12	67%
Non-reversible passives	3/4	75%	3/4	75%
Reversible passives	4/8	50%	5/8	62%
All non-reversible	7/8	78%	7/8	87%
All reversible	9/16	56%	9/16	56%
Gapped	13/16	81%	12/16	75%
Converse relations	5/8	62%	5/8	62%

four sentences described as complement as adjective (e.g. *this man's got more chickens*) and four sentences described as complex complement as adjective (e.g. *this man's got less (sic) horses to feed*).

The sentence comprehension sub-test has been given to MG on several occasions. Bearing in mind the shortcomings aired above what did this test reveal about our subject, MG?

These results show that MG, two years post-onset, like speakers with agrammatism, was performing at chance when the meaning of passives cannot be gained by lexical knowledge alone. Furthermore he was performing above chance on reversible actives, 62 per cent. Testing at seven years post-onset, we find MG performing at chance level on reversible active sentences, above chance on reversible passives but just above chance when these two sentence types are taken together. Clearly, these results do not make sense if we look at the absolute values but more sense if we interpret his performance to be just above chance when NPs in a sentence can plausibly take the thematic role of agent or theme. Alternatively, we may think that the raw scores show that percentage differences between sentence types and change over time is more or less meaningless: on both occasions his scores for active and passive sentences were very similar.

If we look more closely at the performance in the active sentences, it looks as though it is affected by the type of verb in the sentence (table 3.3). We see that he does relatively well when the verbs in both active and passive sentences are non-directional. Verbs that are directional, such as *approach*, seem to cause

Table 3.3 *Scores for MG: active and passive sentence sub-tests from PALPA*

Sentence type	2 years post-onset	7 years post-onset
Actives with a directional verb	2/4	1/4
Actives with a non-directional verb	3/4	3/4
Passives with a directional verb	1/4	1/4
Passives with a non-directional verb	3/4	4/4

more difficulty. Here it is revealed that a lexical factor, that is, the type of verb used, compounds the effect of sentence type. This is a good example of how this test can yield information that adds to our understanding of a comprehension deficit. In this illustration we see that difficulties with sentence comprehension arise from the lexical semantic domain as well as the syntactic. However, the caveat remains that with so few test items it is difficult to be confident of the results and further clinical probes were necessary.

Types of errors are not readily identifiable in this test but when errors involving reverse roles (i.e. selects the picture with the NPs in incorrect thematic role position) are tallied, we find that he is more likely to choose distractors showing reverse roles in passive than in active sentences. One interpretation of these results would be that MG has difficulty in assigning thematic roles to NPs, and if this were so, then this would contribute to his comprehension deficit. The PALPA does not offer any channels for pursuing this line of investigation in either the comprehension or production sub-tests. We must wait until we review the results of an alternative test of sentence comprehension before we explore parsing further.

There is no test of sentence production in the PALPA. The authors refer examiners to a procedure developed by Saffran, Berndt and Schwartz (1989). However, this procedure has been developed to log certain features of non-fluent and especially agrammatic aphasia. It will show certain features of fluent aphasia but, as Edwards (1995) has shown, it fails to capture some important features such as hyper-fluency, logged as the number of utterances needed to produce a sample for analysis. This dimension is pertinent to fluent rather than non-fluent aphasia and may be used as an additional index of severity. But, if we put the omission of sentence production aside, then PALPA can be seen as a useful, although limited, clinical tool. It represents an attempt to use information obtained in experimental conditions and thus reflects a certain state of knowledge. As a consequence, this information was embraced enthusiastically by British speech and language therapists and, to a certain extent, by clinicians in other European countries, although how far the sentence structures tested were relevant to their language is not clear. However, the test's strength is in the number of procedures it contains for examining single-word production. It has to be accepted that what it can reveal about a patient's grammar is limited and confined to what can be gleaned from the sentence-comprehension test.

Testing the production and comprehension of verbs and sentence

Why is it important to look at sentence construction in aphasic speakers? Well, given that aphasia is a language disorder, it would seem to be essential that we look at language production. The production of single words is not necessarily the same as the production of words within sentences, although testing single-word production may throw some light on word-retrieval difficulties, as we have seen above. While testing single-word comprehension and retrieval may reveal the nature of certain deficits of the lexical domain, it can give us only partial information. It is true that most aphasic speakers have problems with recalling words, but the nature of these problems varies across speakers. As we have seen, factors of grammatical word class as well as factors of fluency and familiarity have an effect. Word class is particularly pertinent as there is a major distinction between the two main types of aphasia, fluent and non-fluent, with the former having more difficulty accessing open-class words, such as nouns and verbs, than closed-class words, such as determiners, prepositions, pronouns and auxiliary verbs. Within the open-class category of words, fluent aphasic speakers are thought to have more problems with nouns than with verbs. If we conceive of sentences as being series of words strung together in temporal order, then the ability to produce a sentence could be gauged, perhaps, by an ability to produce single words. If that were the case, then all we would need to do would be to assess aphasic speakers on their word-finding abilities and, essentially, the types of words that can be produced. However, we know that in aphasia, not only is the recall of single words vulnerable but also the ability to construct sentences using appropriate word order and appropriate functional categories. The underlying relationship between the various elements that make a sentence are complex and it is the nature of those different relationships and their different levels of complexities that need to be taken into account in any aphasia examination. It is quite extraordinary that there are few aphasia test batteries that systematically test a range of sentences that are known to be problematic for aphasic speakers.

The Sentence Processing and Resource Pack

We have seen that some of the sentences that are included in the PALPA have structures that have been shown to be problematic for aphasic speakers, that is sentences with reversible NPs. But this test contains a mixture of sentence structures including 'gapped sentences'. The authors state that they have included gapped sentences because 'empty NPs' 'may present difficulties for some patients'. These sentences are included despite the authors' claim on the test forms that they 'do not subscribe' to Binding Theory (Chomsky 1988, Cook and Newson 1996). Because of the time that it takes to design, trial and standardise a test, it inevitably follows that the tests are not able to reflect the most recent research in aphasia or anything like contemporary linguistic theory. Furthermore, they are limited in scope in that they are usually motivated by one area of research and aphasia investigation.

'The Sentence Processing Resource Pack' (Marshall, Black, Byng, Chiat and Pring 1999) reflects some more recent work in the diverse field of psycholinguistics. The pack includes two tests, the first of which tests the ability of a subject to understand reversible active sentences. As with the PALPA, we find that other factors are included in this test. Two types of verbs are specified, 'action' verbs such as *splash, expel, protect* and 'psychological' verbs such as *surprise*. Sentences which have adjectival copular complements such as *the queen is fond of the nun* and sentences which have prepositional complements of the copular verb such as *the boy is behind the bed* are also included. The test has been given to twenty-one non-aphasic speakers as controls but, unfortunately, they did not score at 100 per cent on each section, which creates a problem for aphasic data interpretation.

The second test in this battery is called the Event Perception Test. This taps a level of knowledge about verbs as single words. The task is to select one of two pictures to 'match' the 'event' portrayed in the third picture. The idea is that this will show whether the subject has a correct perception of the activity portrayed. So, for example, given a picture of water being poured from a bucket, the task is to point to a picture that shows water being poured from one container to another rather than the picture of a car being sprayed. The authors claim that that all three pictures share some semantic features but the task is to select a picture that shows the same *event* in both pictures. It is not clear to me how this differs from selecting the two pictures that share the same *verb*, in the example above, *pour*. Clearly, the term *event* is not being used in the way used by writers such as Rosen (1996) or Pustejovsky (1995). In the Marshall et al. test, the *event* is taken to be the activity portrayed by the verb rather than qualities of a verb such as *completion*. There is evidence emerging that people with fluent aphasia find event structure (in the Rosen sense rather than the Marshall et al. sense) difficult to judge (McCann and Edwards 2002). It will be some time before such findings are included in aphasia tests.

A test designed to investigate verb and sentence deficits in aphasia: the Verb and Sentence Test (VAST)

We will now look at a new battery that has been developed to test the production and comprehension of verbs and sentences in aphasia. We will see that the results obtained from this test indicate that similar patterns of results on sentence comprehension may be obtained from fluent aphasic subjects as those we might predict for agrammatic subjects. In a test battery developed first for Dutch aphasic speakers (Bastiaanse, Maas and Rispens 2000) and then adapted and standardised for aphasic English speakers (Bastiaanse, Edwards and Rispens 2002, Bastiaanse, Edwards, Maas and Rispens 2003), the comprehension and production of several different sentence constructions are tested: actives, passives, subject clefts, object clefts and WH-questions. The production tasks involved naming of actions to elicit verbs as single words and within sentences, sentence-completion tasks to elicit finite and infinitive verbs and the elicitation of sentences. The comprehension tasks involve picture selection in response to verbs used as single words and to sentences and making judgements about the acceptability of sentences, some of which are anomalous. Information on frequency and transitivity is given for each verb. The test also includes anagram tasks that may be regarded as involving both production and comprehension skills, for the subject has to understand the sentence constituents if a correct sentence is to be constructed. The level of understanding required in order for the anagrams to be correctly constructed is not known. However, we will look at some results obtained for a group of subjects with fluent aphasia. Passive and active sentences are included in these tasks using reversible and irreversible sentences.

Control data were obtained from a large cohort of non-aphasic subjects (over eighty) during the production of the English version of the test. Each sub-test was given to at least twenty control subjects and all control subjects obtained at least 98 per cent correct response level on all sub-tests.

Performance of fluent aphasic speakers on the test

The Verb and Sentence Test was given to a group of people with different types of aphasia and varying degrees of severity. Consequently not all subjects were able to complete all tests. Results from a subset of the subjects that could be identified as fluent or non-fluent reveal some expected differences between these two types of aphasia as well as similarities that were surprising in some ways. The most obvious difference between fluent and non-fluent aphasic speakers is, of course, output. The fluent aphasic speakers are relatively good at constructing sentences and can speak at a normal speed, with normal intonation for considerable lengths of time. The non-fluent aphasic speakers, on the other hand, speak slowly, hesitantly and with effort. Sentences are ill-formed, often abandoned, leaving single-word and short phrases as the most frequent utterance type. These are diagnostic symptoms used to separate our two groups. So how so do the two groups compare on tests that examine sentence production?

Of the twenty-five people with aphasia who were given the test and could be categorised, twelve were classified as fluent. Three of these, although presenting as Wernicke's aphasics in the acute stage, had recovered to the extent that they could be described as anomic rather than Wernicke's at the time of testing. The other nine matched the criteria for Wernicke's aphasia: they had obvious comprehension problems in conversation, difficulty with accessing content words, made semantic paraphasic errors yet maintained fluent speech. Table 3.4 contains information on all twelve subjects and includes age, years of education, time since onset and the diagnosis that was made available to the examiner.

The aphasic classification given to each subject is based on the diagnoses of the referring clinicians and confirmed by the tester. The separation of the subjects into the two main groups of Wernicke's aphasia and anomic aphasia is based on the perceived comprehension abilities of the subjects and also on their ability to converse in well-formed sentences. Some subjects had better comprehension than is typical in Wernicke's aphasia although that category was the nearest match. Subject JS was referred by his therapist as having conduction aphasia, as she had noted that he had many phonemic paraphasic errors in his speech and she had judged his comprehension to be moderate. However, as can be seen in table 3.5, although this was true for single-word comprehension, understanding of sentences was much poorer. When seen in our clinic, our clinicians confirmed that his copious output was typical of Wernicke's aphasia and, for the purpose of this study, we therefore included his data in the Wernicke's group.

Table 3.4 *Subject information for twelve subjects with fluent aphasia*

Subject	Gender	Age	Years of education	Time since onset (months)	Diagnosis Diagnosis
JoH	M	76	12	63	CVA Wernicke's
MG	M	65	15	103	CVA Wernicke's
MF	F	81	12	15	CVA Wernicke's
IM	M	70	8	7	CVA Wernicke's
MB	F	75	9	6	CVA Wernicke's
EH	F	70	12	3	CVA Wernicke's
JS	M	60	12	6	CVA Wernicke's
MS	F	60	12	15	CVA Wernicke's
DC	M	56	15	9	CVA Wernicke's
DM	M	72	12	12	CVA anomic
CG	M	58	12	20	CVA anomic
TR	M	70	15	17.5	CVA anomic

To a large extent, the classifications used here embrace levels of severity: clinically, the anomic patients present as least impaired and their most obvious deficit seems to be lexical in nature. In contrast, the subjects with Wernicke's aphasia are far less successful at communicating and have noticeable problems with understanding spoken language. Time since onset of the aphasia also plays a part. Four of the Wernicke's aphasic subjects had had aphasia for less than nine months. If their language continues to improve, they may, at a later stage, be reclassified as having anomic aphasia: EH has a relatively high score on the sentence-comprehension test and MS is at ceiling on the verb comprehension test. However, as we will see by looking at some results gained from the VAST, there is considerable overlap of strengths and weakness across these clinical diagnoses.

Understanding of verbs and sentences

First we will consider the data collected from the tasks that examine the understanding of verbs as single words and of sentences. Scores for each test are out of 40. The range of on-aphasic controls scores are shown in table 3.5 below.

These scores show that all of the Wernicke's subjects save one (DC) and one of the anomic subjects made more errors on the sentence-comprehension task than they did on the single-verb comprehension task. The difference is less

Table 3.5 *Comprehension of verbs and sentences: VAST scores for the Wernicke's aphasic group*

Subject	Verb comp: scores out of 40 (control range 38–40)	Sentence comp: scores out of 40 (control range 39–40)
JoH	34	20
MG	38	24
MF	28	20
IM	37	22
MB	33	27
EH	36	30
JS	37	24
MS	40	33
DC	33	35

Table 3.6 *Comprehension of verb and sentences: VAST scores for the anomic group*

Subject	Verb comp: scores out of 40 (control range 38–40)	Sentence comp: scores out of 40 (control range 39–40)
DM	37	38
CG	39	38
TR	37	39

marked for the anomic subject where the ability to understand single words and sentences approaches ceiling for all three subjects. The difference is striking in the Wernicke's group. This group of subjects is clearly better at understanding a verb as a single word than a sentence where most scores are around chance. This holds for MS for whom, you recall, there was some doubt as to whether she could be more accurately described as having anomic or Wernicke's aphasia.

For those with Wernicke's aphasia, it could be that poor performance on sentence comprehension is a reflection of slow language processing: length of sentence is not a factor here. As a group, these subjects were significantly better at active and subject-cleft sentences (where thematic roles are in canonical position) than they were at understanding passive and object-cleft sentences (where thematic roles are not in canonical position). We will look at these results in more detail in chapter 6 when we also consider the types of errors made and endeavour to interpret these findings.

Unlike the Wernicke's group, the anomic group was not noticeably better at understanding single verbs than understanding sentences. For these subjects, the sentence gave, presumably, more contextual clues which, in turn, assisted performance. The errors made in the sentence task, however, did not suggest that mistakes arose from erroneous lexical decisions, as one might predict from the single verb test. They, like the Wernicke's subjects, were more likely to choose the distractor picture depicting the NPs in reverse roles (i.e. an error involving sentence structure) than the distractor picture depicting an incorrect action (i.e. a lexical error).

Production of verbs and sentences

There were three different tests of verbs as follows: (a) production of a verb as a single word; (b) verbs within a sentence; (c) two tests, each of which elicited either (c1) infinitive or (c2) finite verbs. Results from these tests for the Wernicke group and the anomic group are shown in tables 3.7 and 3.8.

The three tests involved the following procedures: when eliciting verbs as single words, subjects were asked to look at a picture depicting an action and name the action (e.g. *mowing*). For the test of production of verbs within a sentence, subjects were asked to look at a second set of pictures and to describe the action using a sentence (e.g. *the man is mowing the lawn*). Finite and infinitive verbs were elicited by asking subjects to supply the missing word in a sentence. Subjects were shown a series of action pictures. Each picture had a written sentence that described the action except that the verb was missing. The verb slot was indicated by dots. The examiner would read the sentence to the subject, omitting the verb, and ask the subject to supply the missing verb. An example of a sentence eliciting finite verbs was *the woman . . . (waters) the garden* and to elicit an infinitive *the man wants (to eat) the dinner*.

Scores shown in tables 3.7 and 3.8 indicate that for five of the ten fluent aphasic speakers for whom we have results (incomplete results for IM and DM) it was easier to produce verbs as single nouns than in a sentence. For the other three subjects, the reverse was true. In each case, the difference is small. Surprisingly, as a group, infinitive verbs were produced correctly more often than finite verbs. Surprisingly, because classically we would not expect the grammatical operation of inflection (however that is conceived) to be problematic for this group of aphasic speakers. This is true for eight of the group of ten (no results for EH and JS).

As we might expect, the data in tables 3.7 and 3.8 show some individual variation. Producing a verb in a sentence was slightly more successful for JOH,

Table 3.7 *Production of verbs as single words and within sentences: Wernicke's group*

Subject	Verb as single words: scores out of 40 (control range 37–40)	Verbs in sentences: scores out of 40 (control range 38–40)	Infinitive/finite verbs in sentences (control range 8–10)
JoH	12	16	3/0
MG	22	18	8/1
MF	35	29	9/5
IM	16	N/A	6/9
MB	29	25	9/0
EH	21	23	N/A
JS	13	9	N/A
DC	27	31	10/8
MS	29	25	10/6

N/A = not available

Table 3.8 *Production of verbs as single words and in sentences: anomic group*

Subject	Verb as single words: scores out of 40 (control range 37–40)	Verbs in sentences: scores out of 40 (control range 38–40)	Infinitive/finite verbs in sentences (control range 8–10)
DM	16	N/A	6/8
CG	28	31	9/6
TR	38	32	9/3

N/A = not available

EH, DC (Wernicke's aphasia) and CG (anomic) than producing verbs as single words. Looking at the different rate of correct elicitation of inflected verbs we find that not all subjects found the non-finite form easier than the finite. Two subjects (IM and DM) showed the reverse pattern with more correct finite verbs than non-finite verbs, although we have to remember that the number of items is small in this test. Unfortunately, we do not have scores for verbs within sentences for these speakers and so nothing more can be said. Notwithstanding these two exceptions, these results show that speakers with fluent aphasia not only have problems with producing verbs as single words, but are all poor at producing verbs in sentences. Producing verbs in sentences was difficult, and whether or not it was more difficult than producing verbs as single words, it would seem that production of a sentence frame, or an attempt to produce a sentence frame, did not make a substantial impact on verb retrieval. There is no evidence here that the assumed intact grammar of these speakers assisted them.

Furthermore, grammar, in particular verb morphology, involving in our test the production of a correctly inflected verb, appeared to hinder verb production. For eight out of ten subjects for whom we have results, production of an inflected verb, a finite verb, was more problematic than production of a non-finite verb. Although this is not classically considered a feature of fluent aphasia, it has been observed in continuous speech, as we will see in the next chapter.

What these results tell us is that, first of all, all the subjects were better at understanding verbs as single words than they were at producing verbs as single words, and secondly, and importantly, that fluent aphasia is not just a manifestation of a lexical deficit. Grammar, in terms of syntactic structure and inflection, did impact on the performance of these speakers with fluent aphasia. Their ability to produce verbs was hindered by sentence structure and inflection.

Summary: limitations of aphasia assessments

In this chapter we have reviewed a number of published aphasia assessments that are currently used in clinical practice and research projects in the UK and elsewhere. All procedures that we have reviewed have limitations of scope and limitations of test construction. Not all have reliable control data; not all relate well to what we know about language: there is no consensus on which variables should be controlled and little information about the internal validity and reliability of test items. Furthermore, there is little consensus on what an aphasia test should be testing. No single test will give all the information that a clinician needs to motivate therapy: no single test score can be used to measure the effectiveness of aphasia therapy. This is not surprising given the complexity of the disorder, but it is a situation that is poorly understood by those who review and fund research. So there is still much work to be done in the area of assessment but, in the meantime, clinicians have to work with the tools available. It is important that they and their co-workers recognise the limitations of their tools as well as recognising the need for a range of assessment measures both to motivate therapy and to act as base-lines for measuring change in language over time.

4   *Connected fluent aphasic speech*

Introduction

In this chapter we will discuss the nature of connected speech samples, their
benefits and drawbacks and whether such data add to our knowledge of fluent
aphasia. We will look at examples of connected speech, noting and examining
errors that occur, and explore some possible explanations for them. The clinical
descriptions of fluent aphasic speech that we examined in the preceding chapters
concentrated on non-segmental and lexical features. We have also looked at
supra-segmental features of fluent aphasia, observing that prosody is said to be
normal while rate of speech is described as abnormal or, by some, hyper-fluent.
However, we have seen that in a study where rate of speech was measured it was
found to be normal. Lexical access is assumed to be deficient and this difficulty
is associated with semantic and phonemic paraphasias as well as the production
of neologisms. In terms of word-processing models, these errors suggest that
deficits are at the semantic and phonological level of representation.

Many accounts of fluent aphasic speech have assumed that syntax is normal
despite the fact that paragrammatism is a defining feature. However, there has
been poor agreement over what paragrammatism is and it is debatable whether
paragrammatism can be considered a syntactic deficit, despite the term. For
most researchers, however, it is the ability to use well-formed sentences that
defines fluent aphasia. Despite the assumption that syntax is intact, there is
plenty of evidence that although fluent aphasic speakers do have the capacity to
use well-formed sentences, they also exhibit problems with sentence formation
and with inflectional morphology. Such errors would suggest that syntax or
access to the grammar is neither effortless nor faultless. We will consider these
points as we look at connected speech.

The nature of speech samples

The data used in studies of fluent aphasia vary from elicited single words
and sentences, under various experimental paradigms, to analysed samples of
so-called spontaneous speech. It is on this last type of data, connected speech,

that we will now focus. Samples of connected speech vary in a number of ways: length, the manner of elicitation and the different methodologies employed in analyses. It is not known whether differing methodologies affect the conclusions but, from what we know to date, it would seem highly likely that this is the case. There is an assumption that connected speech is more naturalistic data than single-word or sentence data collected under experimental regimes and, because it is more naturalistic, it is more representative of the aphasic speaker's language abilities. As we will see, this is not necessarily the case. To the best of my knowledge, all samples are elicited in some way or other. I know of no published data where speech samples are covertly recorded conversations or monologues. There are examples of aphasic speakers talking with relatives, carers, speech and language therapists and other researchers, but in every case the occasion has been structured or at least set up in some way and the speakers know that they are being recorded.

Analyses of connected speech data can be used to explore types of vocabulary and sentences used, discourse and conversational features. The frequency of certain vocabulary items, sentence structures, discourse features can be logged and compared with what is thought to be normal. However, given the lack of robust norms, it follows that there is a fair amount of interpretation about the nature of connected speech data collected in a comparatively naturalistic context just as there is about experimental data, although the manner of speculations differs. Aphasic data must be considered within the local context as well as the more general context of manner of collection. It also follows that the more constrained the elicitation context is, the less is the need for interpretation. However, in constraining a task, we may be not only sacrificing spontaneity but also limiting how far the sample is representative of the speaker's language system.

How to collect a representative sample

The question of the validity of any sample, or how representative it is, deserves noting. A second consideration is the comparability of samples of connected speech collected in different contexts and under different conditions. What level of importance should we attach to data collected from picture description compared to samples of speech collected in sentence elicitation tasks, or compared with monologic samples or samples of conversational speech? These issues are acknowledged in the field. For example, Goodglass has argued that unsubstantiated assumptions may be made about results from restrained tasks, namely that performance in such a task represents language capacity whereas that is not necessarily the case. The problem is acknowledged but to date there is no obvious resolution.

Length

How long should a sample be to be representative? There is no answer to this fundamental question although there are various conventions about the amount of spontaneous speech needed for a meaningful analysis. Brookshire and Nicholas (1994) have suggested that a sample needs to be at least 300 words long, that is, for normal speakers, about two minutes long. Others recommend longer samples: for example Crystal, Fletcher and Garman (1989) recommend samples of about thirty minutes long, or 100 utterances, and Saffran, Berndt and Schwartz (1989) recommend 150 utterances. Immediately, we have not only a large difference of opinion (these recommendations are based on clinical and laboratory experiences rather than empirical evidence), but some practical problems as well. Aphasic speakers vary in their ability to produce 300 words or 100 utterances. A fluent aphasic speaker will be able to produce 100 utterances fairly quickly whereas a non-fluent aphasic speaker would not. This creates problems if we want to have comparable samples for analyses. Secondly, there are various ways of defining the unit of analysis. For example, do counts of words include all paraphasic errors, such as repetition of words and meaningless recurrent utterances such as *you know*? If prosody is part of the definition of an utterance, then, while the fluent aphasic sample will have well-defined prosodic units, the non-fluent aphasic may be analysed as a series of single words.

Setting norms for connected speech analyses

When working with connected speech samples, there is always the problem of interpreting results within what we would like to think are normal parameters. One of the biggest problems an experimenter has to face is how to judge whether aspects of the aphasic data fall into the so-called normal range. In theoretical linguistics, the linguist judges grammatical acceptability using his/her native speaker knowledge of the language or, maybe, by asking other native judges. The same method can be used to identify aphasia errors. Frank or obvious grammatical errors can be easily observed but this provides only part of an analysis. Problems arise when the experimenter wants to look at the sections of errorless speech and to make judgements about frequency of occurrence and distribution within a text, for example, the frequency of questions, complex clauses and so on. It is not always possible to judge what is normal, for normative data are very limited. Some judgements on acceptability are easier. This is the case when context is necessary. For example, the Extended Projection Principle is (in generative grammar) a grammatical property of English whereby sentences have to have a subject although the subject need not be overt. In certain sentence types (e.g. imperatives), the subject may be covert. This is also the case under certain pragmatic conditions such as answering questions or in the so-called diary style. Given a sentence-production task, the aphasic speaker who responds with a subject-less sentence may be responding in the 'diary style' using a covert subject rather than making an error of subject omission. For example, in answer to the question *how was your holiday* the reply *rained every day* is assumed to have a covert subject of *it*. If such a sentence occurs within a conversation or within a narrative, then the appropriacy of the apparent subject omission is more apparent. The surrounding text can suggest whether the lack of a subject is grammatically, or pragmatically, acceptable. What these data cannot adjudicate on is whether a covert subject exists at some level of aphasic grammatical representation.

Effect of context or task

Connected speech samples may be collected in constrained contexts such as storytelling or in comparatively naturalistic contexts such as conversations. The topic given to initiate the sample may affect the type of data gathered. Penn (2000) found that retelling a frightening experience produced consistently longer and richer samples than any of the other tasks she employed, including storytelling and picture description. If comparisons are to be made across subjects and/or time, it is important that the elicitation conditions are kept constant. Those constraints immediately reduce the naturalistic nature of the data.

Assumptions about unobserved phenomena

Another limitation of connected speech data is that, however large the sample, the absence of a structure does not mean that the speaker is unable to make or use that structure. For example, the lack of any questions in the sample doesn't necessarily mean that the speaker is unable to produce questions. There are similar problems with calibrating the frequency of any feature. Unless there are measurements given for data collected from a non-aphasic control group, we cannot say whether the frequency of, say, embedded sentences in a given sample, or of 'repairs' within an analysis of conversation, lies within the norms of non-aphasic speakers. Currently, such data are limited. To try to resolve this, most researchers publishing aphasic data do include some control data but, as we will see, we still need to be careful in interpreting these data. First of all, the number of subjects in a study is usually, with some notable exceptions, small, and, secondly, data are usually collected from one context only. Whereas we can recognise a missing verb or an incorrect inflection, it may be more difficult to judge whether the number of incomplete sentences produced by an aphasic speaker falls outside what we would expect from a non-aphasic speaker.

Connected speech samples and experimental data

Although there are carefully constructed empirical studies that use connected speech data, the experimental paradigm is probably still the preferred method of investigation. These investigations tend to look at small segments of language, single-word or sentence production. During the last few years there have been more studies that apply discourse or conversational analysis. The experimental approach, where small segments of language production or comprehension are examined, is favoured as 'scientific'. Such studies, as well as providing a greater control of variables and constraint of the interpretation of results, provide answers to specific questions. Experimental studies are often devised to explore well-formulated hypotheses whereas studies that have looked at stretches of connected speech have tended to be data-driven rather than hypotheses-driven. Empirical methodology works from hypotheses about the ability to apply rules of the grammar or hypotheses about some assumed language process, and thus the results, it is often claimed, provide a window into the language system rather than a description of surface forms. Tasks are devised to investigate aspects of a deficit that could not be revealed by looking at stretches of connected speech, for example, the ability to understand or produce certain sentence structures. In examining details of a production deficit, a task could be designed to examine the ability to produce verbs. It may be a closure task, a definition task or a picture-naming task. These types of tasks enable a large amount of data to be collected which would be difficult to find in a sample of connected speech. It is unlikely, although not impossible, that the same number and variety of verbs could be collected in connected speech, whatever the elicitation conditions. One important question persists: are the results obtained under experimental conditions truly revealing about the language system and, further, what do they tell us about language that the aphasic speaker has available for everyday discourse?

In one sense, of course, results obtained in experimental conditions are informative about the speaker's abilities, for, as in all testing, the person tested cannot perform above his or her capabilities, provided, of course, the test is well constructed. However, it is the case that, in language testing, because distractions and demands are controlled, the test performance may be better than the performance would be in everyday speech. An aphasic speaker may be much better at producing verbs as single words in response to pictures than at producing verbs within connected speech. Heeschen and Kolk and subsequently Kolk and his colleagues have argued that the differences we hear in fluent and non-fluent aphasic speech arise because of different strategies applied by the two aphasic groups and that, in a constrained task, they sound very similar. Their claims are based on analyses of German and Dutch aphasic data. There are also some limited English data (Hesketh and Bishop 1996, Edwards and Salis in press) that suggest that, like their German and Dutch counterparts, the English aphasic agrammatic speakers adapt their speech according to the degree of constraint of the elicitation task. It is less clear to us that the nature of the task has an equal impact on fluent aphasic speakers. We would, however, expect the aphasic speaker to be influenced by task, although the direction of influence may not always be predicted. The speaker may be aided by the experimental conditions or the reverse may be true. Some aphasic speakers perform less well on elicited tasks than they would in more naturalistic conditions. As yet there are no conclusive findings, partly because the range of features and methods examined vary across studies, so that we are not always comparing like with like. Some studies have found that their experimental data are paralleled by what they find in spontaneous speech and, increasingly, researchers looking at the effect of intervention and working within the experimental paradigm (such as Thompson and her colleagues, for example, Thompson, Shapiro, Kiran and Sobecks 2003) include an analysis of connected speech as part of their base-line measures.

An example of work that compared elicitation techniques is a study by Goodglass and his colleagues where they set out to compare performance in a constrained task with connected speech samples. In one study they compared fluent and non-fluent aphasic speech collected in structured tests and a free narrative task using seven Broca's and seven conduction aphasic speakers (Goodglass, Christiansen and Gallagher 1993). The purpose of the study was to see how far a constrained task would reliably provide information on morphological features of fluent and non-fluent aphasic speech. The investigators found that the production of various morphological structures in the constrained task (third person singular, possessive, plural nouns, auxiliary verbs) was paralleled by the production of the same structures in the free narratives. From this they concluded that, for clinical purposes, the constrained task would give reliable and useful information about a range of bound and free grammatical morphemes a patient could use. Analysis of test material is certainly less time-consuming and easier for clinicians to use. The analysis of connected speech samples is agreed to be very time-consuming and thus resource-hungry. If it can be demonstrated that tasks provide information that can be reliably extrapolated to everyday speech, then this would certainly be the preferred manner of obtaining clinical data on the nature of the deficit and of language change over time. However, it is not clear that constrained tasks always elicit the same type of language that less constrained, connected speech samples would give. Findings are inconclusive. Despite the conclusions of Goodglass and his colleagues in this paper, they show that differences were found and they also note, considering Kolk's work, that different types of constraints might produce different results.

Some examples of connected fluent aphasic speech

With these limitations in mind, we will now look at some connected speech data collected from tasks, storytelling, conversations and so on. First, some examples of elicited sentences. In the task used to elicit them, the person with aphasia is asked to provide a sentence to describe a picture. Examples are given and instructions repeated until the examiner is sure that the subject has understood the task. Such tasks are very common in clinical examinations, in therapy and in some research designs. The advantage is that the examiner knows the target and thus the amount of interpretation needed is limited. However, as we will see from the samples given below, interpretation is still needed and may lead to a range of conclusions about the nature of the language disorder.

Elicited sentences

The examples below (figure 4.1) are from a 63-year-old man who had been aphasic for nine years. His spontaneous speech is typically fluent although containing many well-formed sentences as well as some that were ill-formed. The task was to look at a picture and then produce a one-sentence description of the picture. In this task there were twenty pictures. Examples were given to him before he was asked to produce a sentence. The examiner saw that he understood the task and his understanding of the tasks extended to his predicting that he would have problems with the task, as indeed he did. Below are some examples of ill-formed sentences produced in an elicitation task. The errors made can be viewed in a number of ways. We could conclude, for example, that what we are seeing here is evidence of problems with word retrieval and that the grammar is intact Alternatively, as I will argue, the types of substitutions and omissions in these examples reveal both a lexical and a structural problem.

	Target:	Response:
1.	the man is running	the man running
2.	the man is walking	walking down the street
3.	the man is painting the woman	painting the picture
4.	the boy is hitting the girl	the lady box

Figure 4.1 *Ill-formed sentences produced in an elicitation task*

First the lexical errors. Three of the four lexical verbs, *running, walking, painting*, are produced, while the verb *hitting* is either substituted or omitted. We will return to this point. There are three errors with the NPs: the subject NPs are omitted in (2) and (3) and possibly (4). The NP is in object position, *girl* has been substituted by *lady* in (4). (The picture clearly depicts two children.) It has been suggested to me that the speaker is trying to use a different structure, either by topicalisation (putting the object NP *girl/lady* first), or by passivisation (where the object NP of the active sentence given would be moved to the front of the sentence). However, without further evidence that this is one of the speaker's strategies, I think we can dismiss this suggestion. It is more straightforward to interpret this as a lexical error. The target, *girl*, is not retrieved but a close semantic neighbour, *lady*, is used instead. The speaker then produces a verb but produces *box* instead of *hitting*. This could, like the *lady/girl* error, be an example of selecting a close semantic neighbour (*hit/box*) although, cautiously, it is wise to note that without syntactic structure we cannot judge the grammatical category of *box*. *Box* could, bizarrely, be a noun especially as *box* as a verb has a lower frequency than *hit*. Although frequency has been shown to be a factor in word retrieval for some subjects, it is not uncommon for lexical items with a lower frequency count than the target word to be retrieved. Given that the other verbs *walking, running* and *painting* are produced in non-finite form, then production of a non-finite verb *box* better fits the pattern of these other sentences. There are no other examples here of production of a verb as a noun. Like the other lexical errors, *box* is semantically related to *hit*, the target verb. The other substitution error is semantically related to the target: *lady* > *girl*. Additionally, there are errors of omission: *the man* in (2) and (3) and *the boy* in (4).

These are all the types of errors, lexical errors, we associate with fluent aphasia. We could extend this lexical account and note that there is a word-class effect: substitution applies to nouns and verbs but only the so-called open-versus closed-class words. From this limited sample, our speaker appears to have retained determiners, even when accessing the incorrect noun. But there cannot be a simple open/closed-class lexical explanation, for auxiliaries are also affected, although here the speaker is omitting rather than substituting, and the systematic omission of the auxiliaries is striking. The omission of nouns and the substitution of the lexical verb fit the notion of lexical-semantic deficit but the omission of auxiliaries does not. Furthermore, the omission of the nouns is sentence position linked. Only in (1) does the speaker manage to produce the subject noun; those in subject position in the other three sentences are omitted or perhaps substituted for as in (4) as we have noted above. So, for these few examples, we can see that, even though the task is highly constrained, a lexical account is insufficient to accommodate all these data. We will now consider whether there is any evidence here of a problem with sentence structure, a syntactic problem as well as a lexical problem.

The omission of the auxiliary verb in each example suggests a problem with functional as well as lexical categories. In generative grammar, the auxiliary is generated in the VP node and moves to the INFL node (a functional node) for inflection. In the first three examples there is no tense inflection. The lexical verb is retrieved (at least in three of the four sentences) but none is inflected. A verb is produced but not inflected and we interpret lack of inflection as a syntactic problem not a lexical one. And there is a further problem, with the sentence structure. In (2) there is no subject NP and we could argue that the subject NP is also missing from (3) and (4), although given that the examiner was looking at the same picture, the lack of subject NP could, perhaps, be seen as pragmatically appropriate in all these responses. The response in (1) could be seen as a well-formed NP used to label one feature of the picture. However, it does not fulfil the task requirements *tell me in one sentence what is happening in the picture* and the response suggests that the speaker has difficulties with sentence formation.

In all cases, what the subject does manage to say suggests that he understands each picture, he knows what is in the picture and has some idea of what he wants to say. However, as well as selecting incorrect lexical items and therefore conveying incorrect information (*lady/girl*, *hitting/box*), he omits the auxiliary verb on every occasion, thus failing to describe any of these four pictures using a syntactically well-formed sentence. The omission of the auxiliary verb is strikingly consistent.

Different perspectives yield different interpretations. We will now look at the same data using abstract representations of sentences used in generative grammar. We will adopt the tree-structure representation of the target sentences that gives a visual representation of the assumed abstract relationship between

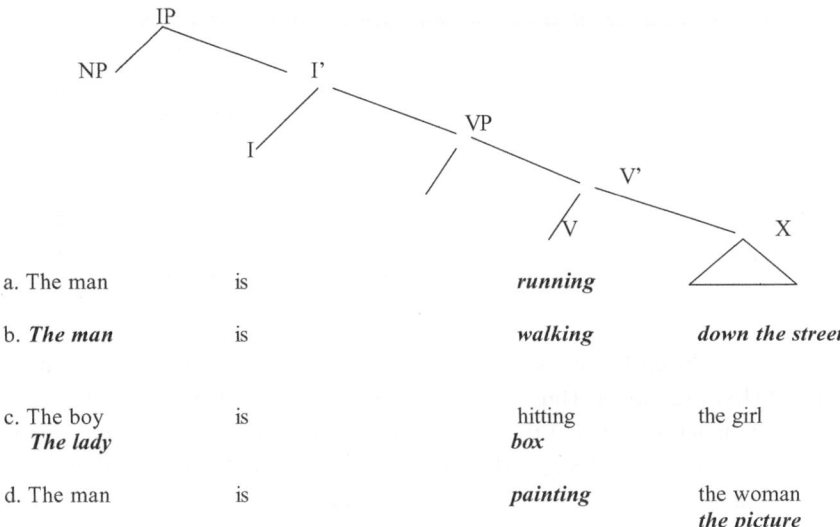

a. The man   is   *running*

b. *The man*   is   *walking*   *down the street*

c. The boy   is   hitting   the girl
   The lady   *box*

d. The man   is   *painting*   the woman
                                                                          the picture

Figure 4.2 *Attempts at sentence repetition: achieved elements in bold*

sentence constituents. Sentences comprise phrases, noun phrases (NP), verb phrases (VP), inflectional phrases (IP) and so on. Phrases can be further broken down into constituents, as represented by branches and nodes. Every branch of the tree represents part of the sentence and every constituent, or node, is labelled according to its category. In generative grammar, not all nodes contain overt material but represent elements of the sentence at some stage of generation. Nodes may be termed *functional* or *lexical*, which roughly equate with open- and closed-class of words. Inflection node may be filled by a morpheme, or an inflected auxiliary verb, as in the examples above. In figure 4.2 the inflection node (IP) splits into I' (I bar) before then splitting into I (inflection) and the verb phrase (VP). Instead of interpreting omission of the auxiliary verb as a lexical problem it could be regarded either as a problem with the functional node I or with the position on the tree. We can illustrate this by using a tree-structure diagram. If we look at this speaker's attempts, and plot what was said compared to the target sentences in terms of hierarchical, syntactic relationships, then the sentences in figure 4.1 emerge in figure 4.2. The tree structure adopted here is taken from generative grammar, for example in Haegeman (1994) and Smith (1999). This tree diagram highlights that, structurally, although errors occur at each node, the first two nodes are more affected than the lower nodes. Starting at the top of the tree, three of the four sentences are either missing the subject NP (in this diagram in what is known as Spec(ifier) of IP) or an incorrect N

Table 4.1 *Distribution of omissions and substitutions in four sentences*

Node	Total target	Correct	Substituted	Omitted	Total correct
Sub. NP	4	2	0	2	2
AUX	4	0	0	0	0
Lexical verb	4	3	1	0	3
Obj. NP	2	1	1	0	1

has been produced for this slot. All four sentences are missing the constituent under I (INFL(ection)). Thus we can see problems located at the top of the tree under IP, under the NP and I'. Three of the sentences have the correct V but in these examples, a non-finite verb, *running, walking*, etc. This fits with the data on test data on finite/non-finite verbs we considered in the previous chapter.

It may be important to make a distinction between substitutions and omissions. Substitutions suggest that the underlying structure is intact whereas omissions *could* suggest that the structure, or node, is not there or, more probably, not available. The distribution of errors of substitutions and omissions is shown in the Table 4.1. Of the first two nodes, subject NP and I, only two out of eight are correctly achieved; six are omitted, which suggests retrieval problems are greater at this level of the sentence. There are no substitutions. In contrast, there are two substitutions and only one omission in the two lower nodes, suggesting a lexical retrieval rather than a structural problem. Thus it looks as though the higher nodes, at least in this task, are difficult to achieve. Lexical items are omitted, so there is no evidence that those nodes have been constructed. In the lower nodes there are two lexical substitutions and no omissions, suggesting the nodes are present and accessible even though they may not be filled correctly.

The speaker clearly understands the task and the pictures but had great difficulty with executing it, producing only two well-formed sentences out of the twenty items in the task. This speaker can produce well-formed sentences in his everyday speech and even in this task he produced two, so it is not unreasonable to claim that these errors reveal difficulties with the task rather than with his grammar. But even if that were true, why is this task, a simple task for any non-aphasic speaker, difficult for someone with fluent aphasia? The speaker understands the demands of the task and can access lexical items, even if they are not the target items, yet has difficulty producing well-formed sentences. The consistent omission of one grammatical element and his obvious difficulty in sentence construction suggests that there is something this task-reveals, over and above lexical retrieval. Although errors of substitution and omission are highlighted in this constrained condition, they also appear in less restrained, connected speech. This speaks to the importance of spontaneous speech data. It acts as a check and a metric by which we can judge the validity of test results in terms of how the speaker can use his aphasic speech. If we find similar errors in spontaneous speech we can be more confident that the tests are revealing something about the language system rather that something about the task. In two studies by Butterworth and colleagues, the speech of fluent aphasic subjects was found to contain a number of inflectional errors. Similarly, Berndt and colleagues found that their fluent aphasic subjects made inflectional errors, suggesting that access to the grammar as well as to the lexicon is damaged.

Why inflectional errors occur

The examples above illustrate problems at the inflection node but we cannot assume that it is missing or not being accessed at all. Although the auxiliary verb is missing in each case, a verb (not always the target verb) is present and has the required aspectual inflection *ing*. Preservation of *ing* while other grammatical morphemes are omitted has been recognised in non-fluent aphasia for many years but it has not, to the best of my knowledge, been recognised as a feature of fluent aphasia. Just looking at this small sample, let us consider some possible linguistic explanations for these data.

Under early versions of transformational grammar, the AUX (auxiliary) node divided into T (Tense) and (modal) (en) (ing) where the brackets signify optional nodes:

$$S \rightarrow NP\ AUX\ VP$$
$$AUX \rightarrow T\ (modal)\ (have\text{-}en)\ (be\text{-}ing)$$
$$T \rightarrow s_1\ present,\ past\ s_2$$

As we can see, tense and *ing* arise under AUX and by affix hopping, *ing* is attached to the lexical verb stem. It is difficult to see how the sentences shown above could be produced given these operations when affix hopping is preserved and AUX is not.

Later development, in the GB framework, the auxiliary *is* is base generated under V and moves to INFL while the verb gains the aspectual inflection of *ing* by covert movement of the INFL to V. The sentence structure is shown in Figure 4.1. The auxiliary verb and the aspectual inflection are still associated to the same INFL node. What is needed here are two nodes: one that is missing or cannot be filled and accounts for the missing auxiliary in these sentences and one that is intact and accounts for the correct *ing* aspectual suffix. There are proposals that the INFL node is split: split INFL hypothesis (Pollock 1989). Although somewhat esoteric, this notion has been central to some explanations of agrammatic production where tense but not agreement is impaired. In order to account for these data, Friedmann used the split infinitive (Friedmann and Grodzinsky 1997) as we will discuss in subsequent chapters. It is interesting to note that it is possible that that split INFL proposal could account for these data in which INFL (the inflection node) is split to form T (tense) and AGR (agreement).

A recent development, over the last five years, in generative grammar has been what is known as Minimalism or the Minimalist Program. In this theoretical development, words are accessed from the lexicon fully inflected and undergo a number of operations whereby elements are merged to form the hierarchical sentence structure. There is no movement as such but items are checked at functional nodes for correct inflection. If there are errors, the sentence crashes and is not produced. Thus the verb plus its aspectual inflection *ing* is selected from the lexicon. In the examples above, three out of the four selections were correct *running, walking* and *painting*. Checking of the aspectual *ing* inflection seems to be functioning for three of the lexical verbs although not for *hitting/boxing* nor for the auxiliary verb. It is missing in each example and therefore this operation must be impaired, at least intermittently. Checking is impaired thus the aphasic utterance is produced. It does not crash before spell-out (the phonological level in processing terms) as it would for the non-aphasic speaker, because now the aphasic grammar allows the ungrammatical sentence through.

Sentence types, well-formedness and complexity

Examination of spontaneous speech data provide important insights into the ease of production and/or the frequency of well-formed components, that is, elements of language. Such insights are not available from experimental data. There has long been an assumption that, given correct lexical access, fluent aphasic speakers will produce syntactically correct sentences. Whereas this might be generally true, it does not address the issue of whether a full range of syntactic structures is deployed or whether the frequency of different sentence types matches that of non-aphasic speakers. There are a number of reports throughout the literature of the last twenty years that demonstrated that neither may be the case. Over twenty years ago, Gleason et al. (1980) noted that their

subjects with Wernicke's aphasia produced a smaller range of syntactic structures compared with their normal controls. In this study continuous speech was
elicited by asking the subjects to retell stories which were illustrated by a series
of cartoons. The performance of three groups of subjects was compared; five
with Broca's aphasia, five with Wernicke's aphasia and five non-aphasic control subjects. Under the heading *syntactic organisation* the numbers of simple
'concatenation' versus 'more complex structures' were compared. The number
of full sentences produced by the Broca's group was considered to be too small
for 'interesting analysis' (p. 379), while the speakers with Wernicke's aphasia
had far fewer complex structures than the non-aphasic speakers. There were
fewer instances in the Wernicke's aphasic speech of embedding by what the
authors term 'temporal conjunction, participle and relative marker' (p. 379). In
their conclusion, the authors note that the syntactic proficiency of fluent aphasic speakers is 'somewhat overrated' and that these types of aphasic speakers
are 'less syntactically diverse than normal speaking subjects' (p. 380). Further
work by other researchers, for example, Goodglass and his colleagues, has confirmed this. In a study examining story retell, abilities of fluent (N = 10) and
non-fluent speakers (N = 10) were compared with normal controls. Goodglass
and colleagues found that the fluent aphasic speakers (in this study the fluent
aphasic speakers had conduction aphasia) had significantly fewer subordinate
clauses in their narratives than the normal controls (p < 0.05). They also found
that the fluent aphasic speakers produced more canonical sentence structures
than the normal control speakers.

   These differences have been replicated in recent studies and are not confined
to English speakers. The restriction of sentence forms in English, Dutch and
Hungarian fluent aphasia has also been noted by Edwards and her colleagues
(Edwards 1995, Bastiaanse, Edwards and Kiss 1996, Edwards and Bastiaanse
1998). There is some suggestion that the language of the speaker may have an
effect on the structures used although the number of our subjects in the 1996
study was small. In these studies, samples of connected English, Dutch and
Hungarian aphasic speech were analysed and proportions of different utterance
types were compared with non-aphasic group data for each language. Comparisons were also made across languages. These analyses showed that, as a
group, the English and the Hungarian fluent aphasic speakers used a smaller
proportion of subordinate clauses than the non-aphasic speakers. The speakers
with fluent aphasia were using less complex language, on this measure, than
their normal controls. However, there was not a significant difference between
the Dutch aphasic speakers and non-aphasic speakers in terms of the proportion of sentence types used in these studies. It was not possible to conclude

how robust this difference was between the language groups, whether it was language specific or an artefact of the coding system. However, the findings of Edwards and colleagues concerning the lower proportion of complex clauses in English is in line with the finding of Goodglass and colleagues discussed above and is also supported by other researchers. Niemi (1990) found that his Finnish aphasic subjects used fewer complex sentences, used a greater proportion of sentences that had canonical word order and less NP elaboration compared with non-aphasic speakers. Similar findings have been found for aphasic speakers of Afrikaans. Penn (2000) reported on a study of the connected speech of seven aphasic speakers from the Cape Coloured Afrikaans-speaking Community. She collected a number of different types of speech samples but the one she chose for analysis was a narration of a frightening experience. In line with other studies, Penn found that her aphasic subjects produced significantly fewer subordinate clauses than the non-aphasic controls. She also found that there were a number of examples of incomplete subordinate clauses that suggested that, at times, the aphasic speakers attempted and abandoned subordination. Although Finnish and Afrikaans differ from English in a number of ways (although Afrikaans and Dutch are closely related), these findings tell us that a reduction in sentence complexity is a feature of fluent aphasia which is not language-specific. The details may vary but the phenomenon is the same.

Analyses of connected fluent aphasic speech

One way of examining language proficiency is to analyse samples of spontaneous speech, quantifying utterance length, types of sentences and diversity of vocabulary through type/token ratios of various word classes, nouns, verbs and so on. In tallying types of verbs, one would count each verb by reference to the root form so that *skip*, *skips* and *skipped* would be tallied as one type but three tokens. Such measures are routinely used in child development and language impairment studies and offer a crude way of making comparisons between normal and non-normal speech. Proportions of sentence types can also be calculated and there are various methodologies being used in aphasia research, although no agreement on which is the most revealing. A detailed methodology developed by Saffran, Berndt and Schwartz (1998) for use with agrammatic production has been used in a number of studies but is not suitable for use with fluent aphasic speech. Edwards (1995) demonstrated that when this method was used with fluent aphasic speech, a large proportion of the utterances needed to be discarded in order to follow the procedures for analysis. Much of the discarded data distinguish fluent aphasic speakers from non-aphasic speakers. No methodology can capture every feature of production and researchers therefore select or develop one to suit their analyses. Hence Thompson and her colleagues at Northwestern University, USA, have developed a detailed protocol for the analysis of connected agrammatic speech. The protocol includes logging details of sentence complexity, verb morphology, verb arguments and lexical details, which are aspects of production that her research focuses on.

Northwestern continuous speech analysis

The Northwestern procedures for examining continuous speech has mainly been used to analyse agrammatic speech. It is a complex research tool but is currently being developed for clinical use and to capture errors in paragrammatic speech and other conditions. Like the Reading analysis we discuss below, it is a grammatical analysis and therefore has not been designed to identify lexical errors although the detailed logging system lends itself to adaptation for this purpose. As with the Reading scheme, features can be added or omitted in the Northwestern scheme to suit the focus of any particular research or clinical investigation.

The coding in the following sample (shown in the square brackets) denotes sentence type, for example declarative sentence [ds], simple sentence [s] or complex sentence [cs]. Sentences are considered flawed [*s] if there are grammatical violation(s) – or errors – shown in the relevant code. For example, if there is an error in verb morphology [*vm3]. Number and type of verb arguments are shown, for example obligatory two place [ob2xy] and how these are realised, for example agent as subject [xs] or object [xo]. A verb morphology index is shown [vmi3] with the number signifying an index of the complexity of the verb's morphology. Tense, agreement and negation are logged as part of the complexity index of the verb morphology. Finally, lexical items are coded. For further details, readers are referred to papers by Thompson and her colleagues (e.g. 1994, 1995 and 1997).

Here is a short passage that has been analysed according to the Northwestern protocol with one amendment. In the example below, sentences that contain lexical errors (as well as those with syntactic errors) are starred even if the syntax is correct. Unintelligible words are signified by X. The full coding is given for completeness although most readers might like to concentrate on the utterances where errors have been identified. The orthographic transcription is followed by the Northwestern coding and then by my commentary on the features of fluent aphasia. The speaker is an elderly man with fluent aphasia describing the Cookie Theft picture from the Boston Aphasia Diagnostic Examination, and the examples have been chosen to illustrate features of fluent aphasia.

1. Northwestern analysis of Cookie Theft picture (BDAE)

1. (uh) we're (in the in the k mp k k n kitchen in) in the kitchen
    [s][ss][ds][e0][copyz][ys][zpp][vmi2][pros][prep][detpo][n]

    The speaker demonstrates that he can see the picture and is aware of the tasks. He produces a well-formed sentence.

2. And there's a lady {f} doing the slowing
    [s][cs][ds][e1][copyp][ys][p][vmi2][ac][ob2xy][*y][#xs][yo][vmi3]
    [conj][pros][det][n][deto][uw]

    Complex sentence [cs] with one embedding [e1] but containing a paraphasic error *slowing* for which the [*y] has been added. Error in y argument.

3. (uh) she's got (the pouring) the plate watching it with with (um)
    [*s][cs][ds][e1][ob2xy][*y][vm3][ob2]["x][*ypron]

    Incomplete complex sentence [*s][cs]; verb used as a noun (the pouring). Error in y argument.

4. The water is (uh) balancing into the sink
    [s][ss][ds][ob2xz][*v][xs][zpp][vmi4][dets][n][aux][prep][detpo][n]

    Grammatical sentence but with paraphasia; *balancing* [*v].

5. The x of the sink [frs]

    A fragment [frs].

6. And the water is pouring (all over the bowing bowing) all over it
    [*s][ss][ds][e0][ob2yz][ys][*zpp][vmi4][dets][n][aux][q][prep][pro]

    Paraphasic errors: the water is pouring out of the bowl/all over the floor.

7. (Uh) she's (got some no cups got) got cups (uh) and (uh) plate
    [s][ss][ds]e0][ob2xy][xs][yo][vmi3][pros][mod][n][conj][n]

8. (Uh) she's (in the wind in) looking out through the window
    [s][ss][ds]e0][ob1x][xs][j][vmi4][pros][aux][ad][prep][det][n]

9. There's some (watches no [w] [gr] [gr s] grass [gr] [gr] grass) grass
   on on the (table) table and there is (some a) a window
   [*s][ss][ds][con][e0][copyp][ys][p][vmi2][copyp][ys][p][vmi2][pros]
   [+q][-det][n][prep][det][n][conj][pros][det][n]

   Potential agreement error between 's and (*watches*)? Target *glasses*
   realised.

10. I can see (uh) x (uh)
    [*s][ss][ds][e0][ob2xy][xs][yo][vmi3][pros][mod][uw]>
11. she's [frs]>
12. I can do that really
    [s][ss][ds][e0][ob2xy][xs][yo][vmi3][pros][mod][proo][ad]
13. I'm doing this bit first
    [s][ss][ds]e0][ob2xy][xs][yo][vmi4][pros][aux][deto][n][q]
14. I get on with that for the moment
    [*s][ss][ds][e0][ob2xy][xs][yo][*vmi2][pros][-aux][prt][prep][pro]
    [prep][det][n]

    Omission of modal *will*.

15. There's a trees
    [*s][ss][ds][e0][copyp][ys][p][vmi2][pro][det] [*n]

    Flawed sentence [*s] agreement error between verb and noun [*n]
    and/or between *a* and *trees*.

16. There's a tree up there
    [s][ss][ds][e0][copyp][ys][p][vmi2][pros][det][n][prep][pro]
17. (Uh) there's [frs]
18. I know that word [s][ss][ds][e0][cxp][xs][p][vmi2][pros][det][n]
19. I've forgotten it [s][ss][ds][e0][cxy][xs][yo][vmi4][pros][mod][proo]
20. (But uh) anyway let's skip over there and get on with the towel up
    there
    [s][cs][ds][con][es][e1][cxs'][#xs][s'][vmi2][obxz][xs][zpp][vmi2]
    [ob2xz][xs][zpp][vmi2][ad][pros][prep][pro][conj][prt][prep][det][n]
    [prep][pro]
21. There's two children
    [*s] [ss][ds][e0][copyp][ys][p]p*vmi1][pros][q][n]

    Agreement error.

22. One of them's sitting on a [t] [ku:l] [tu:l] xx
     [s][ss][ds][e0][ob1x][xs][j][vmi4][q][prep][pro][aux][prep][det][n]

     Incomplete complement of *on*.

23. It's a [frs]>
24. Anyway they've got a (k nki:) cookie jar (with um)
     [s][ss][ds][e0][ob2xp][xs][p][vmi3][conj][pros][mod][det][a][n]
25. Holding with a [s] finger
     [*s][ss][ds][e0][*ob2xy][-xs][-yo][vmi3][prep][det][n]

     Argument violation: requires NP

26. A (uh) biscuit (uh) [ns][det][n]
27. And she's holding her hand up to ask the young girl
     [*s][cs][ds][e1][ob2xy][xs][yo][vmi4][ac][ir][ob2xy][#xs][yo][*z]
     [vmi3][conj][pros][aux][ppro][n][ad][to][deto][a][n]

     Third argument structure of embedded sentence missing: [*z].

28. It's (the the) so that the young man will hold (over her) a biscuit
     down to her
     [*s][cs][ds][e1][copys'][ys][s'][vmi2][oc][ob2xy][xs][yo][j][vmi3]
     [pros][conj][comp][dets][a][n][aux][deto][n][*ad][prep][pro]

     Violation of argument *hold/hand over:* [*ad].

29. Standing to it (uh) [frs]
     KEY: s = sentence; ss = simple sentence; cs = complex sentence;
     ds = declarative sentence; e0 = one embedding; e2 = two
     embeddings; cop = copular verb; ob2 = obligatory two place verb;
     ob3 = obligatory three place verb; op2 = optional two place verb;
     xyz = arguments; xs = agent as subject; yo = theme as object;
     vmi = verb morphology index; pro-pronoun; pros = pronoun as
     subject; conj = conjunction; dets = determiner in subject position;
     a = adjective; ad = adverb; n = noun; aux = auxiliary; * = flawed
     element; # = legally omitted.

In this sample we can see that the speaker tries to describe what he sees in
the picture. In doing so, he uses a number of well-formed sentences and some
complex sentences. However, out of the twenty-nine utterances in this sample,
even if we allow for back-tracking and some mazes, just over half (16) have
errors or are incomplete. What is very obvious in this sample is how sentence

structure is disrupted by lexical errors. Most of these lexical paraphasias involve noun targets, (2) *doing the slowing* when the target was, perhaps, *washing-up;* (9) *grass* for the presumed target of *glass*. In sentence (3) the speaker uses a verb as a gerund, *she's got the pouring* which is similar to the previous error in sentence (2), *doing the slowing*. The proximity of these errors suggests that the episode of word-finding in (2) spills over to the next attempted utterance.

There are agreement errors involving verbs and nouns; (9) *there's some watches;* (15) *there's a trees;* (21) *there's two children*. Whereas the first and last examples may fall within the speaker's dialect, the error in sentence (15) does not.

There are also paraphasic errors involving verbs; *watching it* instead of *washing it; balancing into the sink* instead of *pouring (?out of) the sink; hold over* for, perhaps, *hand over*. In this last example, if this *hand over* was the target, then there is also an argument error, as neither verb allows for a PP *down to her*. However, rather than interpreting this as an error of argument structure, this could be interpreted as a further consequence of verb-selection error. Had the verb been *pass* then a PP is required and *down to her* is legitimate.

Of the twenty-nine sentences, four are complex and, of these, two have errors. The errors in the complex sentences both occur in the embedded sentence, not the matrix. The low number of complex sentences accords with the data discussed above. We can note, though, that in this sample the speaker omits the subject NP in three of the twenty-nine utterances and has errors in the VP in a further three utterances. One of these errors is the omission of the auxiliary verb (14). In this example, we have only looked at some of the features that are logged and readers can see from the array of coding that there are many possibilities.

The Reading aphasia analysis

The starting point of any analysis is to establish what we want the analysis to capture. In the Northwestern analysis, a complex coding scheme has been developed to capture details that have been investigated in Thompson's empirical studies. An analysis for conversational interaction or one developed to capture communicative effectiveness may have a different focus from one developed to capture the features of surface grammar. The focus of the analysis should also motivate the unit of analysis. In conversational analysis, the unit may be a speaker's 'turn' whereas in a procedure developed to capture features of surface grammar, the unit may be smaller, a sentence. In the Northwestern analysis, the unit of analysis is the sentence with all the embeddings.

A different procedure that has been developed to capture features of surface grammar in aphasia is that developed by Garman (1989), Garman and Edwards (hereafter G and E; 1995), Edwards and Knott (1994) and Edwards, Garman and Knott (1995). Their taxonomy and analyses are based on a descriptive surface grammar (Quirk, Greenbaum and Leech 1985 and Quirk, Greenbaum, Leech and Svartvik 1972). It is designed to capture features of agrammatic fluent and non-aphasic speech and uses a grammatical definition for the unit of analysis. This is based on the Text Units as described by Garman (1998). This unit varies from other units of analysis such as 'utterance' where meaning and intonation form part of the segmentation criteria. The Text Unit employed by G and E comprises a verb and associated arguments, and embedded, or subordinate, clauses are given separate codings. The Text Units are classified first of all as: a clause/not a clause. Clauses are units containing a verb and are subdivided into Main (matrix) and Subordinate (embedded) clauses.

Well-formed utterances without a verb are assigned to a Phrasal (multi-word) category and single words to a Lexical (single word) category. Idiomatic phrases, greetings and so on are classified as Minor and there is a further category for utterances that are unintelligible or incomplete. Additional categories can be used if further detail is required. Adjuncts may be segmented from clauses, logged and tallied and types of links between main and subordinate clauses can also be logged and tallied. In the Northwestern analysis, that was developed for the analysis of agrammatic speech, utterances that are not sentences are coded as such but not further subdivided. In the Reading analysis we wanted to log and quantify all utterances, as many fluent aphasic speakers often use proportionately more formulaic speech, incomplete utterance and utterances that are unanalysable because of paraphasia and/or jargon than non-aphasic speakers.

As this is a grammatical analysis, well-formed sentences containing lexical errors may also be logged (as we did above) rather than excluded. Thus a comparison can be made between well-formed grammatical utterances that contain lexical errors and those that are error-free grammatical utterances. In the same way, it is useful to log utterances with inflectional errors. Further error analysis may include distinguishing between the incomplete and unanalysed Text Units and examining the errors contained within those units that are classified as unanalysable.

All these types of utterances are found in non-aphasic as well as aphasic speech, but it is the relative proportions of the categories that differentiate the normal from the non-normal speaker. Non-aphasic, healthy speakers have incomplete sentences, make occasional lexical and grammatical errors, but much less frequently than aphasic speakers. Speakers with aphasia will, generally, have lower proportions of well-formed clausal utterances and higher proportions of incomplete/unanalysed utterances compared with healthy non-aphasic speech. This procedure differs from some others as it is inclusive: all utterances can be included whether or not they are well-formed sentences and whatever the topic. In the Saffran, Berndt and Schwartz (1989) Analysis, comments that are not part of the story retell are neither analysed nor scored. In the Reading analysis, all utterances are included. So, for example, comments about the task or about the problems in word-finding, are all included.

This procedure gives a broad-brush view of connected aphasic speech. Profiles of aphasic speakers can be compiled using the proportions of different Text Units found, and the values obtained by the aphasic speakers can be compared with those obtained by non-aphasic speakers. Profiles can illuminate aspects of production in greater or less detail, depending on the detail of analysis required. For example, comparisons between all types of Text Units, that is, the proportions of main and subordinate clauses, phrasal and lexical Text Units can be computed. Segmentation of continuous speech in this way exposes the proportion of well-formed grammatical sentences, giving an index of grammaticality; the proportion of embedded clauses give an index of complexity, and marking units that contain lexical errors reveal, in a somewhat crude way, the relationship between lexical errors and grammatical structure.

Analyses of continuous speech data

In the final section of this chapter we will look at two examples of spontaneous speech data taken from an elderly man approximately twelve months post-onset. His speech and language therapist had diagnosed Wernicke's aphasia and his fluent output is typical of that syndrome. The following example has been segmented following a simplified version of G and E's procedure. This reduced version is simple and quick to do and offers a realistic analysis for clinical use.

Segmented text is displayed in the first column, comments on errors in the second and the type of Text Unit is given in the third. On first mention, the name of the Text Unit is given in full, thereafter letters denote the type of Text Unit. In this example, adjuncts have not been segmented but incomplete and unalaysable units are given separate codes.

The speaker has been asked to describe a series of cartoon pictures that depict a couple preparing for an ill-fated dinner party.

2. Reading analysis of dinner party theft

Segmented utterance	Errors	Text Unit
1. *and they said*		Main clause (MC)
2. *we're writing*		Subordinate clause (SC)
3. *and so they went the way*	omitted *on their/they* (?)	Unalalysed (UA)
4. *and she was at the boy*		UA
5. *as he was telling it*		SC
6. *and must said*	omission *have* omission argument	Incomplete clause (I)
7. *and they went away*		MC
8. *and come on*	tense/agreement omission PP (?)	I
9. *and they round [crup] at a XX*	unintelligible	UA
10. *and all the sentences wonderful*	omission verb	I
11. *and she brings this lovely p pig back*	incorrect NP	MC
12. *and (and) like that*		Minor (M)
13. *and they go into the thing*	non-specific NP	MC
14. *and the little [chaplin] say*	inflection	MC
15. *oh good morning*		M
16. *and thank you very much*		M
17. *and they went down to the company*		MC
18. *and they went*	omission PP	I
19. *and they didn't say anything*		MC
20. *ah gone*		Lexical (L)
21. *they said*		MC
22. *and they looked out the road*	PP error	I.
23. *and it was a boy*		MC
24. *that's gone*		SC
25. *and he rushed down*		MC
26. *and he [ko]*		I
27. *and he's got*	omission NP	I
28. *he's had [er] little*	omission NP	I
29. *he's laughed at*		I
30. *because he's had a good show*		SC
31. *good*		M
32. *blimey*		M
33. *I think*		MC
34. *he did*		SC
35. *he was a little chap*		MC

In these thirty-five Text Units we find seventeen clausal units although two of these contain lexical errors: (11) and (14). There are four subordinate clauses (2), (24), (30) and (34) although status is dubious given the preceding unit. There is one lexical Text Unit (20) and five minor Text Units that include *oh good morning* and *thank you very much*. The remaining twelve Text Units are either unanalysable, such as (9) *and they round [crup] at a XX* or incomplete, such as (8) *and come on*.

If we look at Text Units that are either logged as incomplete or have missing elements, we find that most are incomplete because the sentence is unfinished. Only two (6) (logged as incomplete) and (10) are clearly missing an element within the sentence although (8) is problematic. If the subject has elided (assuming *they*) from the previous Text Unit, then there is an error of tense: *come* needs to be marked for past tense to agree with (7). Text Unit (10) is missing a copula; (6) lacks a subject although it is linked to the previous clause by the coordinator *and*, so we might assume legitimate ellipsis. Sentence (6) also lacks an auxiliary verb and is unfinished. In all the other incomplete utterances the missing elements are at the end of the attempted sentence; three have an incomplete PP (8, 18 and 22); there is an incomplete final NP in (27) and (28); at (26) there is only a subject pronoun followed by jargon.

This speaker manages to start an utterance but then is unable to complete. If we view this in terms of a tree-structure hierarchy, then we see that the elements that we discussed earlier, the tense node and those nodes assumed to be higher in the tree (and which cause problems to agrammatic speakers), are not so problematic for this speaker. And yet he does not have full control of tense. At least four of these Text Units reveal some problem with tense if we include omission of the auxiliary as in (6) and the copula (which would carry tense) in (10). Text Units (8) and (14) contain straightforward errors. He also has some problem with subject position (as observed earlier): the subject NP at (6) and (8) is not realised. Of the twenty-six Text Units that have the subject position filled, twenty-four of those subjects are pronouns. Where the speaker attempts to retrieve a specific NP, at (10) and (14), he fails to retrieve an appropriate noun. So although most of his errors do occur below tense, in contrast to the elicited examples examined earlier in the chapter, errors are occurring throughout the hierarchical structure. We have to assume, therefore, that the tree is intact. It has not, as has been claimed for agrammatic speakers, been pruned. (This claim will be discussed in the following chapters.)

Clearly the speaker has difficulty with retrieving words from the open lexical classes (including lexical verbs), but it is not possible to say whether the underlying deficit here is restricted to lexical retrieval, for his errors in this sample of spontaneous speech also involve auxiliary verbs and tense. Utterances are ungrammatical as well as lacking in specific information. Thus we see how such data can be revealing about the nature of fluent aphasic speech.

The second example is taken from the same subject at the same time post-onset, this time retelling the Noah's Ark story, a task where he was required to construct a well-known story but without the help of pictures.

3. Reading analysis of Noah's Ark story

Segmented utterance	Errors	Text Unit
1. *well, I am Noah*		MC
2. *and I build the ark*		MC
3. *and we have*		I
4. *what's that*	categorised by intonation	I
5. *he had build the ark*	tense	MC
6. *I can't say it*		MC
7. *have building the ark*	tense	I
8. *that was*		I
9. *oh, I know*		MC
10. *he had*		I
11. *I can't say it*		MC
12. *he has two of the . . . cats*		MC
13. *and two of the dogs*		P (phrasal)
14. *how much he go*		I
15. *you twelve or something*		I
16. *two of the dog*		P
17. *no horses*		P
18. *and four, no five of the (XX) (XX)*		I
19. *five of the horses cows*		P
20. *and five of the*		I
21. *what's*		I

This attempt to retell a story produces a smaller sample of speech than telling a story given a series of cartoons. Using our procedures for segmentation and analysis, we find that only seven of the segmented units can be logged as clauses, all of which are main clauses. There are no subordinate clauses in this sample. Three of the clauses might be viewed as stereotypic, (6) and (11) and possibly (9). As in the previous sample, the speaker has problems with verb morphology. Text Unit (5) and (7) have tense errors, *he had build the ark*; *have building the ark*. Here, there are various possible targets. In the task of retelling a story, we can assume that he was aiming to use a past tense even though he starts off in the first person: *well I am Noah and I build the ark.* Targets could have been *he built the ark* or *he has built the ark*, if he wanted to convey the action was completed. Alternatively, if he wanted to convey a continuing activity, the target may have been *he was building the ark.* He manages none of these. Depending on the target he intends, there are errors of tense and aspect. In two further Text Units, verbs are omitted and hence tense not marked at all; the auxiliary verb *do* in (14), *how much he go*; and the copula in (15), *you twelve or something.*

Of the incomplete units, four are missing a NP following the *verb*, (3) (8) (10) and (21), and two have incomplete NPs. All of these look like examples of lexical retrieval problems, for example where an NP is missing after the verb; (3) *we have*, (10) *he had* and (21) *what's.* The two incomplete NPs can be identified by the presence of the determiner: (18) *no five of the* and (20) *and five of the.* A verb is missing from (14) *does* and (15) the copula *is.* Unlike the previous example, there's no obvious problem with filling the subject position, although careful examination reveals that he uses pronouns in every subject position in this sample.

Two units marked as main clauses, (1) *I am Noah*, (2) *and I build the ark*, are pragmatically dubious. The speaker launches into this task, retelling the Noah's Ark story, by using the first person and present tense, both of which are unexpected and neither is sustained. It could be that this is a strategy to help him with the task but, although found in aphasic data, it is not a characteristic of fluent aphasic speech and he did not use it in the previous task. Gleason and her colleagues examined connected speech collected from ten aphasic subjects. The task was to tell a story given a series of cartoon pictures. They found that there were few instances of direct speech in their control data but more in the aphasic data. Of these, there were many more examples in the Broca's aphasic speech than in the speech collected from the group with Wernicke's aphasia. In the above example, we see that the speaker with Wernicke's aphasia tries to tell the story in the first person and in the present tense, which might be for dramatic effect but were it successful would eliminate the need to mark tense overtly.

These two examples produce rather different pictures of the speaker's abilities. Both samples can be classed as spontaneous speech, but the first was elicited by using a picture description task and the second required the speaker to recall a story. In the first task the speaker's reliance on pronouns might be appropriate in the context of the speaker and listener having access to the same picture. However, this is not the case in the second task and we have seen here that the speaker had difficulty in producing an accurate and appropriate subject

Table 4.2 *Proportions of Text Units in two spontaneous speech samples*

Unit type	Cartoon story	Noah's Ark story
Total clauses	17 (48%)	7 (33%)
Total main clauses	13 (37%)	7 (33%)
Main clauses without error	11 (31%)	6 (28%)
Subordinate clauses	3 (11%)	0
Phrasal	0	4 (19%)
Lexical	1	0
Minor	5 (14%)	0
Unanalysed	4 (8%)	0
Incomplete	9 (26%)	10 (47%)
Total Text Units	35	21

NP and relied heavily on the use of pronoun in subject position. This highlights the speaker's difficulty in retrieving specific nouns.

In table 4.2 we compare the proportions of the text types in the two elicitation tasks. If we take the proportion of clausal structures and proportion of clauses without errors as indicators of well-formedness, we see that the telling of the Dinner Party story, a task with pictures, produces a similar proportion of well-formed clauses to retelling of the Noah's Ark story. There are 31 per cent and 28 per cent well-formed units, respectively. But the Noah's Ark task elicited more phrasal units, perhaps because the story permits listing of animals, but there is no obvious reason why retelling a story would not elicit subordinate clauses. So we could conclude that the second task, the task without pictures, is the harder task for this speaker. The same is true if we look at the proportion of unanalysed and incomplete utterances. If we take the unanalysed and the incomplete text units together, the first task yields 34 per cent and the second 47 per cent. This means that nearly a third of the units in the first task, and nearly half in the second, were not well formed. Using this index, the second task again looks the more difficult task. Both samples reveal a moderate to severe difficulty in spontaneous speech arising from difficulties with word-finding, sentence structure and verb morphology. One parameter of severity is a comparison with other aphasic speakers. A second would be with non-aphasic speakers. We can compare the proportions of Text Units displayed in the table 4.2 with some normative data collected by Edwards and Bastiaanse (1998). They looked at the continuous speech of forty subjects, twenty were

Table 4.3 *Two samples of continuous fluent speech compared with control data: values as % of total number of text units in sample*

| | Aphasic subject | | Controls (N = 10) | | |
| | | | Retell event | | |
Text unit	Story retell + picture	Story retell	Mean	SD	Range
Main clause	37	33	42.9	6.92	32–54
Subordinate clause	11	0	18.5	4.74	14–27
Total clauses	48	33	61.5	9.28	49–78

English speakers and twenty were Dutch. In each language group, ten were fluent aphasic speakers and ten acted as control subjects. Control subjects were spouses or close friends of the experimental subjects and similar (although not matched) in age and education. The subjects were asked to talk about the onset of their aphasia, or (for the non-aphasic speakers) the last time they had visited a hospital. Each sample, that is from each control subject, comprised 100 Text Units, longer samples than those discussed above, but the segmentation and analyses were the same. It was found that the English fluent aphasic speakers, although able to use main and subordinate clauses, used significantly fewer, as a group, than the control group. In table 4.3 we can compare the above samples we have discussed with the control values gained in the 1998 study. This comparison shows that the proportion of main clauses, in both samples, falls within the control range. However, the proportion of subordinate clauses falls outside the control range for both samples. The low proportion of subordinate clauses affects the proportion of all clauses and we see that this falls just outside the control range for the first sample and below one standard deviation for the second task, the story retell without picture. These findings for our subject MG are in line with the findings for the English group reported by Edwards and Bastiaanse and discussed above.

The analyses examined here confirm the presence of a word-finding problem but additionally suggest that the problem is manifested in different ways, depending on sentence position. In subject position, the speaker is more likely to use a pronoun than a proper noun and this was true for both samples. Lower in the tree hierarchy (sentence structure), following the verb, this speaker will not fill the slot with a pronoun but struggles to select a suitable NP or PP. Lack of success leads to incomplete units, which is especially marked in the

Table 4.4 *Reading analysis of Cookie Theft (shown above in 1. Northwestern analysis)*

Text Unit	Story retell + picture	% of total TUs	Mean	SD	Range
	Aphasic subject		Controls (N = 10) Retell event		
Main clause	21	47	42.9	6.92	32–54
Main clauses without errors	11	30			
Subordinate clauses	2	0.6	18.5	4.74	14–27
Total clauses	23	66			
Phrases	2	0.6			
Phrases as adjuncts	3	0.9			
Incomplete/unanalysable	10	26			
Well-formed clauses + phrasal + adjuncts	18	47			
Total number of Text Units	38		61.5	9.28	49–78

second sample. In this small sample where 47 per cent of the units are incomplete, seven of the ten incomplete units had unfilled NP slots following the verb. Given this difficulty, it is not surprising that fewer complex sentences are achieved although, as discussed in this monograph and elsewhere (Edwards and Bastiaanse 1998), lexical accessing will not explain all the difficulties with sentence construction.

Comparing two analyses

Different analysis will produce different results but the differences should not be very large. Earlier, we looked at the Northwestern analysis where, on a sample of twenty-nine utterances (or units of analysis), we found that approximately 50 per cent of them were well formed. If we submit the same data to the Reading analysis the first difference we find is that the Reading analysis results in more units of analysis, thirty-eight compared with twenty-nine on the Northwestern. The proportions of the Text Unit types arising from the Reading analysis are shown in table 4.4. We see that, although the data have been segmented in a different way, we still get more or less the same proportion of well-formed sentences (47 per cent). What this analysis reveals over the Northwestern analysis is separate units for subordinate clauses, phrases and adjuncts. If we want to go further in the analysis we can see the proportion of Text Units that were well-formed clauses is 30 per cent which is lower than the 50 per cent of well-formed utterances logged in the Northwestern analysis. The information remains essentially the same, namely that a large proportion (between one third and a half) of this speaker's utterances are not well formed. The difference arises in that the matrix clause of a sentence is not always intact. Both methods show that the proportion of embedded sentences (Northwestern) or subordinate clauses (Reading) are low in these data compared with control data. Furthermore, the comments given alongside these analyses show that sentences are disrupted by problems with lexical retrieval, verb inflection and the realisation of all verb arguments.

In all these samples, there are examples where missing NPs are missing verb arguments. In the Northwestern analysis we can see this in utterances (10) *I can see (uh) X (uh)*. In the Reading analysis of the Dinner Party Theft there are examples in (27) *and he's got* and (29) *he's laughed at*. And there are further examples in the Noah's Ark story retell: (3) *we have*; (10) *he had*. So the consequence of lexical retrieval difficulties can lead to failure to complete the verb's argument structure and, where the argument is obligatory, this results in an ungrammatical sentence.

Summary

There are strengths and weakness for most methods of analysing aphasic speech. These analyses confirm that there are problems with lexical retrieval, verb inflection and verb argument structure, and that these problems occur in spontaneous speech as well as in test conditions. Furthermore, the analyses provide a way of quantifying not only the errors but the level of reduction in certain complex structures. The analyses we have looked at provide a way of logging and quantifying features of fluent speech and comparing them with the same features in non-aphasic speech. We see that lexical retrieval problems impact on grammatical structure and that, further, there are problems with verb morphology, especially tense marking. These errors may be infrequent and noticed only when a sample of speech is examined.

5 Non-fluent and fluent aphasic speakers: what are the differences?

Introduction

In this chapter we will review some studies that have highlighted the differences between fluent and non-fluent aphasia. A description of non-fluent aphasia was given in chapter 1, largely based on work of Goodglass and his colleagues. Clinically, fluent and non-fluent aphasias sound different but the boundaries between these two aphasia types are not always clear and not all patients can be clearly identified. Over the past twenty years or so, there have been a large number of studies that have set out to investigate specific aspects of agrammatic speech, some of which have included fluent aphasic subjects as one of the control groups. These studies have been based on the premise that some division of aphasia types is justified and that what is required is a more precise definition of the nature of aphasia, especially aphasia arising from lesions in the anterior areas of the fronto-temporal region. These lesions are typically found in the area known as Broca's area but may extend into adjacent left frontal peri-Sylvian cortex (Ullman, Corkin, Coppola et al. 1997:273). The subjects under scrutiny are variously referred to as Broca's aphasics, non-fluent aphasic or agrammatic subjects. Remember that all agrammatic individuals have Broca's aphasia but researchers do not regard Broca's aphasia as inevitably synonymous with agrammatism. The varied use of these terms is not always justified and the debate about what does and does not qualify as agrammatic is unresolved and tangential to our purposes.

Linguistic accounts of aphasia and agrammatism

There have been numerous studies of non-fluent rather than fluent aphasia and numerous papers on agrammatic comprehension, many of which start with an overview of the field of research (e.g. Druks and Marshall 1995, Grodzinsky 1995, Berndt, Mitchum and Haendiges 1996, Blumstein, Byma, Kurowski, Hourihan, Brown and Hutchinson 1998). Despite, or maybe because of, extensive investigations there remain long-held opposing views on the underlying nature of the deficit. Below we will examine some accounts and work on the assumption that characteristics of aphasic symptoms, and specifically of agrammatism, can be explained by evoking specific linguistic frameworks. Within these accounts, it is held that linguistic characteristics arise because of damage to the underlying linguistic architecture associated with distinct cerebral loci. In fact there are few who now hold that the deficit is one of loss of representation, rather that the condition arises as a consequence of deficient access to that representation or a deficiency in specific grammatical operations. Under either interpretation, we would not expect to see the same linguistic characteristics in fluent aphasia as in non-fluent aphasia. Essential features of agrammatism output include reduced sentence structure and difficulty accessing functional rather than lexical categories, or closed-versus open-class words. In comprehension, a specific pattern of deficit arises in which canonical sentences (classically active sentences), but not non-canonical sentences (classically passives), are understood above chance. However, this distinction has faltered as it became apparent that (a) some patients with unquestionably agrammatic output have not shown the hitherto defining comprehension deficit and (b) some non-agrammatics, patients with unquestionably fluent aphasia, show similar comprehension deficits.

There are relatively few accounts of agrammatism that draw on linguistic theory but these have been very influential in the field. Some, with the clearest linguistic motivation, set out their accounts and then predict what aphasic data would look like if the accounts were correct. One of the best-known accounts of agrammatism within this paradigm is that developed by Grodzinsky and his colleagues. I will spend some time reviewing these accounts of agrammatism as they provide a distinctive view that there is an underlying deficit that is unique to agrammatism in the syntactic representation. If the accounts prove to be true, then it follows that the account cannot be applied to fluent aphasia, in particular to paragrammatic speech we find in Wernicke's aphasia.

There are two main theories, the *trace deletion hypothesis* in its various forms, that accounts for deficits in sentence comprehension (Grodzinsky 1990, 2000a and b, Balogh and Grodzinsky 2000) and the *tree-pruning hypothesis* that accounts for errors in sentence production (Friedmann and Grodzinsky 1997, Friedmann 2000). These accounts work within two frameworks. Firstly, the framework of aphasic syndromes: there is an underlying assumption that there is a psychological reality to the notion of aphasia syndromes. For Grodzinsky, there is overwhelming evidence of the reality of at least one syndrome and that is agrammatism. While recognising individual variation, or even because of individual variations in severity, Grodzinsky considers that it is important to abstract away from the differences found between subjects and concentrate on commonalties. He considers that the 'traditional classification [is] not only justified but also useful for theory construction' (Grodzinsky 1991:563). Even when empirical evidence shows that maybe there are not the predicted differences between syndromes (Balogh and Grodzinsky 2000), people working within this paradigm point out that features of surface grammar may arise from different underlying causes. Researchers working within the classical syndromic framework argue that not only are there differences in how aphasic speakers sound or how they perform on comprehension and production tasks but there are also specific linguistic accounts of why language behaviour differs among aphasic patients. Furthermore, linguistic differences are the consequence of different lesion loci.

The second framework for these theories is the linguistic framework of generative grammar. Using Government and Binding Theory, Grodzinsky and colleagues recruit concepts of *trace, co-indexing, movement, empty categories* and *hierarchical relationships* between *phrase structures*. These relationships are conceived and visualised as *tree structures* as we saw in the previous chapter. Some of the linguistic details of the explanations about the nature of agrammatism may look somewhat dated to theoretical linguists, perhaps because theories trickle down rather slowly from the linguistic field to aphasiology. Theories, as applied to aphasia, are certainly simplified but we can assume certain lasting fundamental concepts of generative grammar, especially the notions of a mental lexicon and a grammar, that is a set of rules for constructing words and sentences. Grammar is conceived as a mental organ with dedicated operations that can account for, *inter alia*, different sentence structures. These operations are at an abstract level, known as D-structure. Grammatical operations at this level can account for similarities between sentences that, on the surface (S-structure), look very different. These concepts have been used to account for the association between sentence structure and aphasic performance in sentence comprehension and production tasks. There is an eagerness in the field not only to relate this work to that of other researchers working within the same theoretical framework but also, inevitably, to refute the claims made by those not working within this framework. A small industry has thus arisen that generates studies that support linguistically based interpretation of the aphasic data and studies that claim to disprove these interpretations.

Comprehension deficits and agrammatism

While Broca's aphasia was thought to be a deficit of output only, that is, a modality-specific deficit, the lack of comprehension deficits was accommodated. In the mid-1970s, Caramazza and Zurif (1976) demonstrated that people with Broca's aphasia did have comprehension deficits that seemed to be associated with certain syntactic structures. We will review these in detail in the next chapter, as these studies laid the foundations of many claims about the contrastive nature of comprehension loss in fluent and non-fluent aphasia. Once comprehension problems in Broca's aphasia were exposed, a new view arose that Broca's aphasia resulted from a central syntactic deficit, but it soon became clear that there were major problems for this view. If Broca's aphasia, or agrammatism, resulted from a damaged grammar, rather than from a deficient output only, then there would be a need to demonstrate that there was parallelism between the output and the comprehension deficits. If the grammar, the central knowledge of language, is damaged then both speaking and understanding should be deficient in similar ways. There would be a need to demonstrate what Grodzinsky (2000b:74) has described as an overarching agrammatism. This point has not yet been reached.

A large number of studies focusing on sentence comprehension have led to an almost universal agreement that there is a group of patients, usually known as agrammatic, who can understand certain types of sentences above chance and others only at chance. Furthermore, this pattern of sentence comprehension deficit separates agrammatism from fluent aphasia, specifically conduction and Wernicke's aphasia. Classically, the two exemplar sentence types that can differentiate populations are active sentences, *the tiger chased the lion*, and passive sentences, *the lion was chased by the tiger*. The difference in comprehension ability of these sentence types is only found when the NPs are reversible, that is when either of the two NPs in the sentence can plausibly take the theta roles of agent or theme. Theta roles are the relationship the NP has with the verb, that is whether NP is doing the action, or is the theme of the sentence, or experiencing the action, or is the goal and so on. NPs keep their theta roles even when moved. So, in the second example above, *the tiger* has the theta role of agent: it is doing the chasing; *the lion* has the theta role of theme: it is the one being chased. This remains the case even though *the lion* is the subject of the sentence in the passive example above. *The lion* is still the one being chased. When the two NPs are not reversible, then agrammatic listeners are able to access meaning by relying on their lexical knowledge. In a task where an aphasic listener is required to select a picture to match the sentence or verify a sentence, such as *the apple was eaten by the boy*, the non-animate first NP *apple* is not assigned the agent role incorrectly. The listener knows that apples don't eat boys, so, providing they have adequate access to the meaning of the word, that lexical knowledge will be sufficient for accessing the meaning of the sentence. When, however, the NPs are interchangeable, as in *the lion* and *the tiger*, the aphasic listener is not able to assign the theta role correctly. Both NPs, *the tiger* and *the lion* are animate and therefore either can be the agent in the sentence. Either of the NPs can, plausibly, perform the action of the verb.

Studies have demonstrated that problems with understanding passive sentences extend to other sentence structures. It has been found that object-cleft sentences, *it was the tiger the lion chased*; object relatives, *the lion that the tiger chased killed the cub*; and certain questions, *which lion did the tiger chase?*, are problematic. These sentences have similarities at D-structure level of representation. The robust pattern of sentence comprehension has led to a number of linguistically motivated explanations as well as those that claim that the deficit is not within the grammar per se, but in the interface between syntax and meaning. The listener has problems mapping the meaning to the structure.

We will consider some studies that are motivated by a framework of generative grammar. Here it is assumed that in sentences where one or more constituent has been moved from one sentential position to another (at an abstract level of representation), there is a trace (that is an abstract link between the old and the new position) that is necessary for interpretation of thematic role (Crain, Ni and Shankweiler 2000:295). Grodzinsky and colleagues claim that, in agrammatic aphasia, traces are deleted and therefore the agrammatic listener is not able to use linguistic processes to interpret the sentence and relies on non-linguistic heuristic strategies for interpretation. When lexical information is not sufficient to disambiguate the sentence, *and* theta role cannot be assigned to the first NP of a sentence, then the listener assumes that the first NP is agent. This works for active sentences (even though there is subject movement and trace, which, presumably, is deleted). The aphasic listener assigns theta role of agent to the first noun, not through trace but by a non-linguistic strategy: first NPs are likely to be agents. As there is no competitor for this role, the sentence is interpreted correctly.

(1)   **Non-aphasic theta role assignment**
        the tiger   chases   the lion
        agent   theme

(2)   **Aphasic theta-role assignment**
        the tiger   chases   the lion
        agent   theme

Grodzinsky and colleagues claim that the difficulty arises with non-canonical sentences, that is where the NP with the *theme* role has been moved to become the first NP of the sentence rather than the second. In normal speech, the NP following the passive verb would be assigned theta roles by the passive *by*:

passive verbs cannot assign theta roles. The NP in subject position would be assigned a theta role by *trace*, that is the link between the moved NP and its D-structure or original position where it was assigned theta role by the verb. In agrammatism, movement of the NP occurs but there is a lack of trace, a defective trace or, in Grodzinsky's words, deleted trace. Lack of trace leads to non-assignment of theta role. The listener, who has no access to trace, has no linguistic means of assigning a theta role to the first NP. In English, all NPs need a theta role. As agents most commonly occur at the beginning of the sentence the aphasic listener therefore assigns the role agent by means of what Grodinsky calls a referential strategy. 'Assign a referential NP a role by its linear position if it has no theta role' (Grodzinsky 2000b:80). However, the second NP of the sentence is assigned agent role by the passive *by*. The listener now has two NPs competing for the role of agent and selects at random. When asked to state who is doing the action, that is which NP has the agent role, he guesses. Guessing leads to an at chance performance on comprehension tasks.

An illustration of non-aphasic (3) and aphasic (4) role assignment is given below for a passive sentence. Intact trace is indicated by the connecting line below the sentence. The dotted line indicates that trace has been deleted.

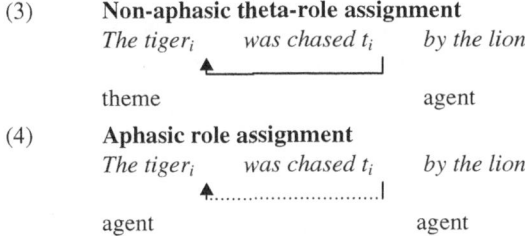

(3)   **Non-aphasic theta-role assignment**
       The tiger$_i$ was chased t$_i$ by the lion

       theme   agent

(4)   **Aphasic role assignment**
       The tiger$_i$ was chased t$_i$ by the lion

       agent   agent

An object-cleft sentence has a different surface structure from a passive sentence but here, as in the passive construction, there is movement at D-structure: the NP that has the theme role has been 'moved' to a position in front of the agent:

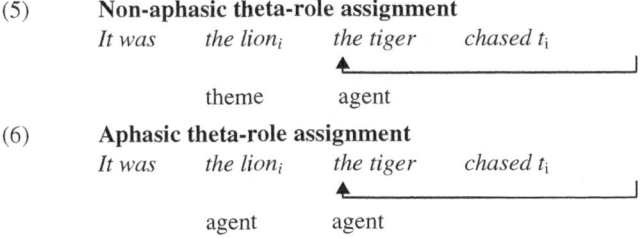

(5)   **Non-aphasic theta-role assignment**
       It was   the lion$_i$ the tiger   chased t$_i$

                  theme   agent

(6)   **Aphasic theta-role assignment**
       It was   the lion$_i$ the tiger   chased t$_i$

                  agent   agent

So although the passive structure and the object-cleft structure look different in their surface form, they share certain syntactic properties, movement and trace, and thus aphasic performance on one type of sentence predicts performance on the other. This was found to have been the case for Broca's or agrammatic aphasia in a large number of studies. It is not thought to have been found in Wernicke's or conduction aphasia, although recent studies are challenging this finding.

There are variations on this explanation. Hickok (1992, 1993) and Hickok and Avrutin (1996) have suggested that object gap sentences contain two NPs that do not receive thematic roles. They claim that the linguistic properties of these sentences differ *qualitatively* and it is the additional linguistic complexity rather than loss of trace that is problematic for aphasic listeners.

How safe are the claims about agrammatic comprehension?

This interpretation of results is held firmly by some researchers despite the fact that we know by looking at a range of studies, and by day-to-day clinical practice, that not all Broca's or agrammatic patients conform to this pattern and that the pattern is not exclusive to Broca's aphasia. Berndt, Mitchum and Haendiges (1996) surveyed studies on agrammatic comprehension that had been published between 1980 and 1993 and looked at comprehension performance on active and passive sentences. They analysed sixty-four data sets obtained from forty-two different agrammatic subjects. The difference between the number of data sets and the number of subjects arises because some subjects are used in a number of different studies. They found several different patterns of results. Although they found that twenty-three samples, or 36 per cent, of the analysed data sets were in line with the agrammatic pattern of actives being understood significantly better than passive sentences, other patterns emerged. In another third of the data, both actives and passives were understood better than chance and in the final third of the data sets, performance on actives was not better than chance. So it was a mixed group. The group that performed well can be considered to be representative of agrammatic patients who have very mild comprehension disorders, and it has been recognised that not all patients who have agrammatic output have agrammatic comprehension. In contrast to this, some agrammatic patients included in this survey seem to have very severe comprehension problems if they were at chance on both actives and passives. This still leaves a group that conform to the pattern of good understanding of active sentences and understanding of passives at chance – what the proponents of the syndrome would recognise as 'true' agrammatics. What still has to be resolved is why fluent aphasics also produce this pattern of sentence comprehension deficits if their underlying syntactic structures and processes are intact. We will discuss this further in the next chapter.

Linguistic accounts of production deficits in agrammatism

If underlying syntactic processes are defective or under-specified in Broca's aphasic comprehension, we would expect to see similar problems in production, that is, Grodzinsky's over-arching agrammatism. That is, unless we assume there is a separate grammar for output and input, which is not argued for. In fact passives, object clefts and so on are not found in Broca's aphasia. As things stand, Friedmann and Grodzinsky have proposed two separate accounts for comprehension and production data. They have proposed a linguistic account of agrammatic speech, again couched in the language of the Government and Binding accounts of Universal Grammar. They illustrate their account by reference to syntactic trees that have hierarchical relationships that are visualised as nodes and branches, as is standard in generative grammar. In their account, the characteristics of agrammatic speech, poor sentence structure and imperfect realisation of functional categories, can be explained by the truncation of the syntactic tree. Not all nodes are equally impaired but are preserved or impaired according to the position on the syntactic tree (Grodzinsky 2000b:75). In their model, an agrammatic speaker has access only to the lower branches of the syntactic tree, specifically those elements that are below tense. Thus the nodes of inflection (IP), complementiser (CP) and associated specifiers (SPEC) are not available. This offers an explanation, they claim, for why agrammatic speakers make errors in tense and negation and cannot form complex sentences. They cannot access the complementiser phrase and thus cannot make complex sentences, e.g. *I think that the cat is hungry*, nor use embedded clauses, e.g. *I saw the cat who bit the man get run over*. They have difficulty with wh-questions where the wh-question word is in CP, e.g. *what did the cat eat?*

This is what an agrammatic syntactic tree might look like for a simple declarative sentence, with the elements that are accessed/spoken in bold font, and those which are assumed to be in the target sentence but not accessed in italic font. The elements at the bottom of the tree are specified while those towards the top are not.

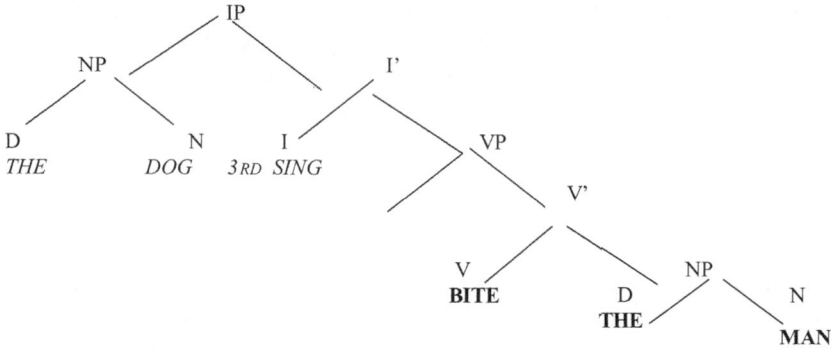

For the target sentence *the dog bites the man* the agrammatic speaker would not be able to access the higher nodes of the tree. They may be able to produce *bite* and *man* but would probably fail to say *the dog*. Furthermore, although they may access the verb *bite* they would not be able to inflect the verb and thus would produce *bite* instead of *bites*. They might be able to access the final noun *man* and, according to this theory, would realise the determiner. So we can list the features of this assumed agrammatic sentence thus: the subject NP and the verb inflection are omitted because they are above V in the syntactic tree. In this model the determiner in the second NP would be realised.

We have seen that fluent aphasic production is often in complementary distribution on the syntactic tree. We have seen that the fluent aphasic speaker may achieve the higher nodes but then fail to produce the post-verbal arguments. However, it is not possible to claim that the lower nodes of the syntactic tree are underrepresented in fluent aphasia, as the fluent speech we have examined in the previous chapters contains well-formed sentences as well as some ungrammatical and incomplete sentences. In addition, there are many utterances where the lower but not the higher nodes are specified. Diagrammatic representation of syntactic relationships highlights some differences in the production data. We will return to a more detailed discussion of syntactic trees in fluent aphasia below.

Tree pruning

Friedmann and Grodzinsky (1997) use a split IP with T(ense) and Agr(eement) as shown on the hierarchical syntactic tree below. The adoption of Pollock's (1989) split inflection hypothesis was contingent on Friedmann's observation that in her Hebrew data (collected from one speaker), inflection but not agreement was compromised. This was confirmed in later data collected from a group of Israeli and Palestinian Hebrew aphasic speakers. The authors claim that the agrammatic production results from the tree being pruned at T node, and that renders all nodes above T under-specified. Their agrammatic syntactic tree would look something like this where IP node has been split into Tense TP and Agreement AP:

All the nodes above the line would be impaired and therefore not available and would account for lack of complex sentences, lack of auxiliary verbs and tense errors. This explanation alone, while accounting for many of the features of agrammatism, does not capture them all. For example, omission of determiners does not fall within this account except for NPs in subject position. Under Friedmann's model, determiners would be realised below, but not above T, although observations of agrammatic speech suggest that determiners are at risk wherever they occur in the tree. I'm not aware of any clear data that can resolve this for English aphasia at present, although some recent work suggests that there is a difference in production of determiners in German, depending on where the determiner appears in the sentence. Grodzinsky (1990) has already proposed an account that suggests that determiners are not realised as they are non-lexical nodes: in agrammatic speech lexical nodes are filled while functional nodes are not. Whichever way the data fall out, it can be seen that these theoretical accounts amount to powerful linguistic explanations of the features of agrammatism.

There are some other accounts that differ from those described above, but we have spent some time with Grodzinsky's account as it is probably the best specified and, although widely criticised, is also very influential. Other researchers, notably Ouhalla (1993) and Hagiwara (1993, 1995) have separately produced rather similar accounts. Ouhalla claims that functional categories are deleted (which in effect results in nodes above T being deleted), while Hagiwara links her account of lack of functional categories to the syntactic hierarchical relationships between elements. These last two accounts deal with the reduction of 'function' words in agrammatic speech while Grodzinsky's observation of non-realisation of functional categories in combination with Friedmann's tree-pruning hypothesis accounts for most, but not all, of the linguistic features of agrammatism.

Comprehensiveness of the account

None of these accounts deals with the slow and effortful characteristics of agrammatic speech but that can fairly easily be put aside by one or two possible explanations. The first resorts to a different domain, that of motor control. Agrammatic speech is associated with lesions in Broca's area that border part of the cortex known as the motor strip. This part of the frontal lobe is associated with motor control; it controls movement of the body's muscles. It is thought that at least some of the difficulty with speech production is motoric in origin and is described by some as apraxia of speech. The second explanation (and these explanations are not exclusive: both conditions may be present) is that given that agrammatic speakers have relatively good comprehension, then it is reasonable to assume that they will be monitoring their output. Monitoring of errorful output may cause slow delivery of speech. There is some support for this idea from two quarters. Kolk and his associates have suggested that the difference between fluent and non-fluent aphasic output arises as the non-fluent speaker, but not the fluent speaker, recognises the danger of making errors and therefore slows her speech, while the fluent speaker does not have that control and thus makes errors. The agrammatic speaker *adapts* to the new reduced level of competency while the fluent speaker does not make the same adaptation. Butterworth and Howard advanced a similar idea to account for the errors made by speakers with fluent aphasia. They suggested that some cognitive device of *control* was deficient in fluent speakers. They observed that all the types of errors made by fluent aphasic speakers were made by normal speakers, but the frequency of errors was much greater in fluent aphasia. Their study did not include agrammatic speakers, though, and thus we can only speculate that if a *control* device is part of the speaking process or mechanism and is impaired in fluent aphasia, then it could also be impaired in non-fluent aphasia; but Butterworth and Howard have nothing to say on this.

Both these theories have been discussed earlier in the book. While they are not adequate to account for fluent aphasia, they do offer some simple accounts for what we might refer to as the articulatory aspects of agrammatic speech. This still leaves us with some characteristics of agrammatism not accounted for. Notably, there is the lexical accessing problem and within this, the phenomenon that verbs are more likely to be problematic than nouns. One reasonable way to deal with all the data would be to offer a syntactic account, the tree-pruning hypothesis, to account for poor sentence structure, reduction of complex sentences and difficulty with inflection. Additionally, the notion that lexical but not functional nodes are realised is needed, particularly the non-realisation of determiners below the tense node. Furthermore, there needs to be a further *additional*, although *associated*, deficit within or accessing the mental lexicon. This would need to account for the difficulty in accessing nouns which, although not as compromised as verbs, are not accessed normally. Friedmann confronts some of these problems and adds an additional detail to the tree-pruning hypothesis to account for the verb problem.

She claims that verbs are difficult for aphasic speakers to access if they are inflected. She notes that there is a difference between accessing inflected verbs and verbs that are in their base form. If the syntactic tree is pruned at tense (IP or INFL) then speakers will not be able to realise verbs that are inflected as the inflection node is above the verb node on the syntactic tree. There is some support for this claim from Bastiaanse and van Zonnenfeld (1998). They found that Dutch aphasic speakers were better at using verbs that were in their base position (sentence final) than using verbs that had been moved and were inflected (those in the matrix clause). Finite verbs in matrix clauses are moved to become sentence second while verbs in matrix clauses that have auxiliary verbs remain sentence final. It was found that Dutch agrammatics made errors on the finite, moved verbs but not the infinitives. This leaves the need to account for the superiority accessing nouns compared with verbs.

A fluent/non-fluent distinction?

Do these findings separate Broca's aphasia from Wernicke's? Largely they do, at least for production. We have seen that, by and large, sentence structure is often intact in fluent aphasia and that errors occur at the beginning of a sentence (the top of the syntactic tree structure) as well as the end of sentences (that is towards the bottom of the syntactic tree). Unlike the classic agrammatic speaker, we cannot draw a syntactic tree structure that is typical for paragrammatism. It is less clear that there is such a distinction between the nature of the sentence-comprehension deficit in these two types of aphasia, although comprehension deficits are more severe in fluent aphasia and encompass lexical as well as sentence difficulties. But there is accumulating evidence that a similar pattern of sentence comprehension can be found in fluent and Broca's aphasia and we will return to this below and in the following chapter. There is also some evidence that verb access may be compromised in fluent as well as Broca's aphasia. We have already reviewed some data collected by Edwards and Bastiaanse that showed that at least some fluent aphasic speakers had a less diverse range of verbs compared with normal speakers. In a more recent study, Bastiaanse and Edwards (2004) found Dutch and English aphasic speakers to be better at completing sentences with infinitive verbs than inflected verbs. Furthermore, and importantly for this chapter, this was true for non-fluent and fluent aphasic speakers across a range of severity. All four groups, English and Dutch fluent and non-fluent aphasic speakers, were less successful at accessing finite verbs than non-finite verbs in a sentence-completion task. To date, no coherent explanation of these difficulties has been worked out.

Some experimental studies

We will now examine a few on-line studies starting with some conducted by Zurif and his colleagues (e.g. Shapiro, Gordon, Hack and Killackey 1993. Zurif, Swinney Prather, Solomon and Bushell 1993, Zurif and Swinney 1994, Swinney and Zurif 1995, Zurif and Pinango 2000). They have used on-line procedures to investigate sentence processing, the ability to recruit long distance dependencies, gap-filling and the processing of verbs and argument structure. In the sentence-processing tasks, they examine a range of syntactic representations and operations, such as movement, trace and co-indexing. These researchers, like Grodzinsky, also work within the general framework of Universal Grammar and are largely influenced, at least to date, by the Government and Binding and the Principles and Parameters frameworks (Shapiro 2000). Both research groups are making similar assumptions (to those discussed above) about underlying linguistic representations and grammatical operations that are implicated in aphasia, although some interpret their results as arising from processing difficulties rather than under-specification of the syntactic tree, nodes or grammatical operations. They have investigated the abilities of people with fluent and non-fluent aphasia to process certain contrasting sentence structures such as actives, passives, object clefts and subject clefts and have investigated the processing of verbs with a range of argument structures. On-line investigations giving reaction times of normal subjects have, they claim, established the psycholinguistic reality of certain linguistic constructs: gaps, co-indexing and, to a lesser extent, movement. They have then applied these experimental techniques to aphasic subjects in order to explore these linguistic operations.

Antecedents

Zurif, Swinney and their colleagues have conducted a series of experiments comparing the abilities of fluent and non-fluent aphasic speakers on tasks which investigate linking of antecedents and trace. In these studies, subjects listen to sentences and, at a certain point, have to make a lexical decision about a word that is flashed onto a screen. Different sentence constructions have been used to examine the relative influence of syntactic structure and lexical semantics. Sentences used include subject-cleft sentences as in (7).

(7)   *The man liked the tailor $_t$ with the British accent ^{1} who ^{2} $_{(t)t}$ claimed to know the queen.*

assumed co-indexing

Priming was examined at two points in the sentence indicated by superscript 1 and 2. Subjects would listen to the sentence and have to make a lexical decision, that is whether the word they saw on the screen was a real or non-word. They were quicker at making a decision if the word they saw was related to the antecedent. In example (7), they would be quicker deciding that *needle* was a word than they would be judging *elephant*. However, this effect was found only where the assumed gap co-indexed by trace to *tailor* occurs, and shown in the above example by the subscript $(_t)$. Co-indexing is indicated by the subscript $_t$. Thus *the tailor* would prime words like *needle* but only if trace is available.

These are known as cross-modal tasks as they involve both auditory and visual activity. Lexical decisions are required at two points in a sentence. One point is where there is assumed to be a gap that is linked to a noun that has appeared earlier in the sentence (an antecedent), indicated by superscript 2 in the above example. The other point is not in a gap position (indicated by superscript 1 in the above example). Some of the words in the lexical decision task are semantically linked to the antecedent, others have no semantic link. The assumption is that if the trace between the gap and the antecedent is intact, then the antecedent can act as a prime, and words that are semantically associated with the antecedent will be judged quicker (on the lexical decision task) than those that are not semantically linked. This is indeed what Zurif et al. (1993) and Swinney, Zurif, Prather and Love (1996) found for the normal subjects.

However, they did not find that this was the case for listeners with non-fluent aphasia, which suggests that either trace was deleted (supporting Grodzinsky's claim) or the 'automatic processing' (Zurif 1995:390) was not available to non-fluent subjects. In contrast, and of interest to us, is that the Wernicke's subjects in these experiments showed the same pattern of activation as the normal controls, although performance was much slower. That is, Wernicke's subjects were able to reactivate antecedents, via trace in this interpretation. When these antecedents were semantically linked to the lexical item, then the antecedent acted as a prime and the decision that this was a real word was made quicker than when there was no semantic association between the antecedent and the lexical target. Thus the authors conclude that, in Wernicke's aphasia, trace is intact but not in Broca's aphasia. These data fit very nicely with the claims of Grodzinsky discussed above.

It may seem strange that the Wernicke's subjects, who we assume have problems with comprehension and specifically comprehension of words, were primed. In this and other tasks, we can observe that the on-line performance of the Wernicke's subjects suggests that they have not lost semantic entries of lexical items otherwise they would not show priming. However, typically, Wernicke's subjects will show some loss of lexical semantics in off-line tasks. This suggests that the central semantic representations for the lexicon can be intact, although accessing this information is problematic.

Verb processing

We now turn to look at some similar studies that explore both verb processing and sentence processing in order to see what they reveal about language-processing abilities in Wernicke's aphasia. We will start with some studies by Zurif and his colleagues that have used the on-line experimental paradigm described above. The first study is by Shapiro, Gordon, Hack and Killackey (1993) and was designed to explore the real-time access of verb-argument structures in a group of Broca's aphasic and a group of Wernicke's aphasic subjects.

The authors report on three experiments, all of which involved cross-model lexical decision tasks. The verbs used in the first experiment were contrasted on the active/passive dimension. In addition, they contrasted verbs that allowed a single, two-place argument (Agent Theme) and verbs that, as well as allowing two-place arguments, also allowed three-place argument structures (Agent

Theme Goal): transitive versus dative verbs. In a separate analysis, within the first experiment they also compared two-complement verbs (allowing agent-theme and agent-proposition) with verbs that allow four-complement structures: agent-theme, agent-proposition, agent-exclamation and agent-interrogative.

The task in the experiments was to listen to sentences over headphones and, on seeing a word flashed onto a screen, decide whether it was a real word or a non-word. Words appeared just after the verb and further away from the verb, down-stream, allowing for calculations to be made on the effect of position within the sentence. Reaction times were recorded. It was found that both normal control subjects and the Broca's aphasic subjects reacted differently to the different types of verbs with significantly longer reaction times for dative than for transitive verbs but no difference in sentence types. This difference was not found for the Wernicke aphasic subjects. They did not show longer reaction times for dative sentences regardless of whether they were active or passive sentences.

A similar pattern was found in the two further experiments performed where the first set comprised object- and subject-cleft sentences with dative or transitive verbs and the second set had object- and subject-cleft sentences with two versus four complement verbs. The verb *know* takes various complements: a NP *I know Jane*; a complement clause *I know (that) he will phone me*; an object clause *I know what I want*; expletive *I know how to do it*. In these circumstances, unlike the normal controls and the Broca's subjects, the subjects with Wernicke's aphasia did not show longer reaction times to the more complex sentences. In the discussion, the authors claim that the Wernicke's subjects 'did not show sensitivity to the thematic properties of the verb' and suggest that the subjects either have a problem representing the verb's thematic information within the lexicon, or have difficulty accessing that information (p. 441). These results hold true for the groups studied.

The groups are quite small and it is therefore reasonable to look to see what the individual variation within the Wernicke's group is. The four Wernicke's subjects used in the Shapiro et al. paper were diagnosed on a series of clinical tests. Three of the four were described as having 'empty speech'; one was described as having fluent speech but with considerable word-finding difficulties. On a preliminary test given for active/passive sentence comprehension, two performed at above chance on both active and passive sentences, although performance was worse on passives; one subject performed at chance on all sentences; one subject performed at chance on active sentences and above chance on passive sentences. That is, none showed the classic agrammatic pattern. In the experiments, one of the Wernicke's subjects showed the expected transitive/dative distinction in active sentences and two of the subjects showed the distinction in passive sentences (p. 433). We also learn that one of the Wernicke's subjects showed the normal two-complement/four-complement distinction. Additionally, we are told that two of the Wernicke's subjects showed the transitive/dative distinction with cleft-subject sentences and two showed this distinction with cleft-object sentences. Finally, we are told that three of the Wernicke's subjects yielded faster reaction times in the padded cleft-subject sentences with dative verbs than they did for those sentences with transitive verbs. The two-complement verb sentences provided faster reaction times than the four-complement sentence (although this was not significant) and padded subject-cleft sentences yielded faster reaction times than padded object-cleft sentences, although down-stream rather than in the immediate vicinity of the verb.

What does this tell us about processing in Wernicke's aphasia?

Wading through these complex results one is left with various impressions. First of all it is clear that, taking the group results, there is a nice distinction between the way in which the Broca's subjects are reacting on on-line tasks and the way in which the Wernicke's subjects react. However, further details are not so clear and it is rather debatable whether the results for the fluent aphasic subjects that were lacking in clear patterns can be taken to indicate any-thing about Wernicke's aphasia per se. For some subjects, on some tasks, the reaction times showed similar patterns to the normal and Broca's subjects. Unfortunately, the subjects who showed these trends are not identified in the paper so we do not know how random these results were. Had it been one or two of the subjects showing these trends throughout the experiments, then conclusions about the differences between the two aphasia groups would be less secure. One has to assume that these results were spread across all four subjects for the authors to reach their conclusions about Wernicke's aphasia. We are told, however, that three of the four Wernicke's subjects were the same subjects used in another study by Zurif et al. (1993). In this study, the same experimental paradigm was used, that is, a cross-modal lexical decision task with calibrated reaction times. This time, the focus of study was on the ability of aphasic listeners to reactivate the antecedents of NPs in sentences containing *trace* as discussed above.

Shapiro et al. note that their findings concerning the activation of possible verb argument structure contrasts with the findings of the Zurif et al. (1993) in which priming was shown in sentences designed to test the presence of *trace*. In this set of experiments, it was the Wernicke's aphasic subjects, not the Broca's subjects, whose reaction patterns mirrored the normal controls. However, in all these experiments the Wernicke's subjects had much longer reaction times than those with Broca's aphasia who in turn had longer reaction times than the non-aphasic controls.

These two sets of results persuaded the authors to claim that in on-line sentence-comprehension tasks, Wernicke's aphasic subjects do not have access to the 'set of lexical-conceptual roles' associated with verbs. A separate set of experiments led them to conclude that Wernicke's aphasic subjects do have access to trace and the associated antecedent. Thus a double dissociation is claimed. Wernicke's patients are seen to have lost access to what they term a 'lexical' procedure, that is accessing all of a verb's possible argument structures, but retain the syntactic processes that allow them to co-index NPs with their antecedents.

Some further complications

In the studies viewed above, the subjects were required to listen to a sentence through headphones and make a lexical decision about words flashed onto a screen, that is they were required not only to use both hearing and visual modalities but to read the single-word stimuli. Blumstein et al. (1998) used a different method, an auditory lexical decision paradigm in which both the sentence and the lexical decision target were presented auditorily. The authors claim that their method reduces the attention load, that the subject is not required to change modalities and the procedures represent more closely normal language comprehension (p. 151). Furthermore, their method removes the need to read, a skill often damaged in aphasia. There were six subjects with Wernicke's aphasia in this study, all diagnosed by a series of clinical tests. The results of these experiments turn out to be at odds with the results of Zurif et al.

In the Blumstein experiments, the subjects were required to listen to sentences spoken by a male voice and judge whether a word spoken by a female voice was a real or non-word. Sentences were described as 'filler-gaps' and were of four different types; wh-questions, relative clauses where the relative clause was the subject of the main verb, relative clauses as objects and embedded *wh*-questions. The lexical stimuli consisted of related and non-related words. The assumption is that reaction will be quicker to the related word, that is the word related to the moved constituent in the gap sentences because of trace. There was also a set of control sentences that did not contain gaps. In the non-gap sentences, where there is no trace, there will be no significant reactivation, whether the word is related or unrelated, as there is no trace to link it to the moved constituent. An example from Blumstein et al. is as follows:

(8)   which   gun   did the trash collector find – in the alley?
             hat   *shoot*

Shoot is related to the first sentence but not to the second. The assumption is that *gun/hat* has been moved from the slot where the lexical stimuli *shoot* is heard. If the sentence starts *Which gun* then the reaction time involved in deciding that *shoot* is a word will be faster (because of the trace between the gap and the NP) than the reaction time for *shoot* if the sentence starts with *which hat*. The fact that these differences are only significant in the sentences that have trace is crucial for the conclusions. If the reactions are not significant, then it could be argued that there is a general activation from the first NP.

Unlike Zurif and colleagues, Blumstein and colleagues found that their Broca's subjects did show a significant difference between the control and the experimental conditions. Thus the subjects reacted faster in the lexical decision task when the target word was related to the moved constituent than when it was unrelated. The difference in reaction time was significant in the experimental conditions (where there were gap constructions) and not in the control sentences (where there were not gaps). All sentences were matched on a number of important features such as length, word frequency and the pragmatics of the sentences. The authors interpret the significant faster reaction time of the Broca's subjects as evidence that there was semantic reactivation of the filler at the gap sites. This is at odds with the findings of Zurif et al.

A second difference in their findings, and of interest here, is that in the Zurif et al. experiments, the Wernicke's subjects were able to show reactivation at the gap site. This finding led to the conclusion above that Wernicke's aphasic subjects did maintain the syntactic structure, in this case trace, while it was lost or unavailable in the Broca's subjects. Blumstein and colleagues suggest that there are several potential reasons why the results of her group do not replicate those of Zurif's group. The first is methodological. They point out that there were variations in reaction times amongst the Wernicke's subjects and that the group was very small: four in the Zurif study and six in the Blumstein et al. study. These factors could be responsible for the non-significant results. The second explanation put forward raises the possibility that performance may vary according to modality. It could be that the Wernicke's subjects in this experiment were poorer at dealing with the auditory stimuli. The cross-modal design may, in fact, have enhanced these subjects' performances. The third explanation offered concerns lexical memory. They suggest that results may arise because of an inability to maintain the semantic representation of the prime word until the semantically related target appeared. The final explanation is syntactic: the lack of significantly different reaction times may arise because of a 'deficit in associating traces with their antecedents' (p. 101).

When performance in Wernicke's aphasia resembles that in Broca's aphasia

If we take these results with those from the above studies we can begin to see that some Wernicke's subjects behave very much like Broca's subjects on some tasks that have been designed to explore syntactic operations. To complete this section we will now look at two further studies, both on sentence processing where no difference was found in the performance patterns of Broca's and Wernicke's subjects. In a study by Balogh and Grodzinsky (2000) it was found that, contrary to expectations, the Wernicke's subjects performed in the same way as the Broca's subjects on sentence-processing tasks. (Our observations here, are, once again, restricted to sentence processing in Wernicke's aphasia. To the best of my knowledge, there has been no attempt to apply the *tree-pruning hypothesis*, to Wernicke's aphasia.) The theory motivating this study is the Trace Deletion Hypothesis, as described above, and its successor, the Trace Based Hypothesis.

In this study, the authors investigated the understanding of four sentence types: active (*the man pays the woman*), agentive passive (*the man is paid by the woman*), short passive (*the man is paid*) and quantified passive (*every man is paid by the woman*). The results show that both the agrammatic subjects and the subjects with fluent aphasia performed above chance on the active and quantifier passive sentences but at chance level on the short passive and agentive passive sentences. The ability of the agrammatic subjects to comprehend the quantified passives looks, on the face of it, a violation of the Trace Deletion Hypothesis (TDH) but Balogh and Grodzinsky explain the results using the Trace Based Hypothesis which has been developed from the TDH.

They claim that the subjects' success on the agentive passives with quantifiers, *every man is paid by the woman*, is because of the quantifier and that this is consistent with the TBH. This revised account now takes note of D(iscourse)-linked phrases and non-D-linked phrases. Referring to Pesetsky (1987), they note that non-D-linked phrases are quantifiers and adjoin to S' while D-linked *wh*-phrases are not quantifiers. They then claim that cognitive strategies and in particular the default strategy of the TDH apply only to referential properties.

The default strategy applies when the comprehender cannot assign case to the moved NP because trace has been deleted but only if the NP is referential. Non-referential *wh*-expressions are outside the scope of the strategy. So, in movement-derived structures with agentive predicates, chance performance will only be predicted if the moved constituent extracted from the object position is referential. If the moved constituent is non-referential, then performance should be at normal levels even though it has passive structure (Balogh and Grodzinsky 2000:91), because the subject will not apply the non-linguistic strategy. So far so good. The next move in this argument is more problematic. The authors say 'because the strategy (whose interaction with the rest of the thematic representation brought about by guessing) is now absent, . . . the patient *can infer the correct thematic representation from the available information*', (my italics). Their results confirm their predictions but what they do not do is to demonstrate what those representations are and how they are now available. Is the NP *every man* assigned a thematic role and if so by what means? It is not clear how the non-referential status of the NP *every man* can overcome the loss of trace which, by his own accounts, is essential for theta role assignment of moved NPs. Does the aphasic listener assign agent by non-linguistic heuristics as was claimed in the earlier accounts for above chance performance for actives? Or, conversely, if trace is preserved in non-referential expression, why should this be?

The background to this study has been given because of the interesting results. The researchers found that the subjects with Wernicke's aphasia obtained the *same* results as the Broca's subjects. They were above chance on the active sentences and the passive sentences with quantifiers but, like the Broca's subjects, they were *below* chance on the agentive passives. Balogh and Grodzinsky say that although they predicted that there would be a difference there is, in fact, no reason why the comprehension performance of these two groups of patients should not overlap. They note that these similarities need not undermine the notion of syndrome as there are many well-documented differences between the two groups (p. 101). The nature of the comprehension disorder is poorly understood, that is true, but what is interesting here is that the performance of this particular group of Wernicke's aphasic subjects is so similar to that of the Broca's subjects. A lexical explanation cannot account for their failure to understand agentive passives while succeeding on passives containing a quantifier.

The work reviewed above has suggested that traces are activated in Wernicke's aphasia but not in Broca's aphasia although the evidence in this study is at odds with earlier findings. Could it be that the elegant explanation developed to account for agrammatic aphasic individuals' difficulties with certain sentence structures is not confined to those patients who have sustained lesions within a circumscribed region of the left frontal lobe, as claimed by Grodzinsky (2000b:101)? Here, Balogh and Grodzinsky suggest that recent findings are beginning to emerge to suggest that there is some involvement of the temporo-parietal areas in syntactic processing although the nature of the disruption, they claim, is likely to be different.

The findings reported here would not surprise clinicians who observe that their Wernicke's patients often make very similar errors to their Broca's patients on comprehension tasks. Some examples from clinical data are given in chapter 2. Once again, there is a possible problem with subject selection and with the size of the group. In the Balogh and Grodzinsky study, there were four subjects described as Wernicke's aphasics. However, the behavioural information given about these subjects is sparse, although details are given about site of lesion. Three of the four are described as being fluent and anomic; two are described as having paraphasic errors in their speech. No information is given about the presence or extent of a comprehension problem, a defining feature of Wernicke's aphasia. The method of the study involved the subjects' making truth judgements on sentences that followed short stories. Given the examples, it is hard to imagine that many patients with Wernicke's aphasia could cope with this experimental design, certainly not if their comprehension deficit is severe. In our clinical work we have found that moderate to severely impaired patients with Wernicke's aphasia tend to have a 'yes' bias in their responses and are therefore considered unreliable on truth-judgement tasks. One can assume, therefore, that the subjects in this study had mild comprehension impairments. It may be that two of the subjects in this study could be more accurately described as anomic and two as having conduction aphasia. It could be that more putative cases of Wernicke's aphasia would have produced the expected performances on the test sentences. However, given the subjects used, we would not predict that the same pattern of comprehension deficit would be found in the two experimental groups, as there are several studies where the performance of anomic patients has been found to differ from that found in Broca's aphasia.

Sentence types and subject types

On the other hand, many other researchers do not find evidence for a distinction between these two types of aphasia, at least on sentence-processing tasks. Claims have been made that there are certain features about sentence structures that make them difficult to process and that these features have a larger effect than patient type. Furthermore, these difficulties arise because the aphasic subjects have diminished processing capacities and their insufficient resources result in failure to comprehend the complex sentences. This view is in contrast with that of Grodzinsky, especially, but also somewhat different from Zurif and colleagues who think that the double dissociations that are found support their view that there are specific and dedicated resources responsible for the different performances on different sentence types. For Grodzinsky, these difficulties arise because of loss of linguistic operations: Zurif and colleagues (e.g. Zurif and Swinney 1995) remain neutral on this point. Further, we have seen above that Blumstein et al. suggested that their small subject group might have contributed to the lack of difference they found between their Wernicke's and Broca's subjects.

Caplan, Waters and Hilderbrandt (1997) looked at sentence comprehension using a picture matching task. They had previously used an enactment task and part of the motivation for this study was to try and replicate their findings using different procedures. In the experiment discussed here, fifty-two aphasic subjects participated in a picture-selection task. Nine of the fifty-two are described as fluent aphasics and this group included patients with anomia, conduction aphasia and Wernicke's aphasia. As with the Balogh and Grodzinsky study, the group was mixed and we might expect that comprehension abilities would vary within this sub-group. Ten examples of ten different sentence structures were given. All sentences were semantically reversible. There was one foil for each sentence. Performance was measured in terms of syntactic complexity and of number of propositions. Cluster analyses were performed to establish subgroups of patients. None of the sub-groups defined included patients with 'particular clinically defined types of aphasia' (p. 547) and the authors conclude that clinical classification is not a good guide to sentence comprehension (p. 552). The authors found that, overall, patients showed sensitivity to two aspects of sentence form. They found that canonicity of order of thematic roles played a part, with active and subject-cleft sentences easier than passives and object clefts. Secondly, they found the presence of a second verb or proposition added to the difficulty for their subjects. The findings applied equally to the fluent as to the non-fluent subjects.

Unresolved issues

Both Zurif's group (and to a lesser extent Grodzinsky's group) have contrasted the performance of agrammatic speakers with that of speakers with fluent aphasia as a way of specifying agrammatism, highlighting the unique nature of agrammatism and confirming the status of a syndrome. In many investigations there are differences in behaviour that seem to confirm the uniqueness of syndromes. In the discussion of results, these researchers have explored possible reasons for the differences and speculated why these differences might occur. But differences have not always been found. Similarities, they claim, do not demonstrate that errors in agrammatism and in fluent aphasia arise from the same underlying disorder. However, there is a need to provide answers to why similar errors should be found in aphasia associated with different lesion loci. There is growing speculation that there may be an involvement of the temporoparietal areas in syntactic processing or that lesions involving neural networks cause widespread damage and not just to the functions associated with site of lesion. This is entirely consistent with evidence we have discussed in chapter 1 and is in line with results obtained by researchers who have not found evidence for a sharp divide of language behaviour based on loci of lesions. In research projects, care can be taken to choose subjects that are highly representative of a particular syndrome. Even so, the results don't always turn out as predicted, that is, with results differentiating between agrammatic and other types of aphasic subjects. The performance of fluent aphasics may match that of the agrammatics or not differ significantly.

Some studies on agrammatism are motivated to validate the syndrome as well as to refine the definition of the syndrome and include fluent aphasic speakers either as control subjects or as a means of contrasting agrammatic speakers' abilities with those of other aphasic speakers. Results obtained by these controls provide information on specific aspects of fluent aphasia. Experimental studies focus on limited phenomena, as this method of study, if well executed, requires considerable resources. The best-controlled studies tend to look at a select range of linguistic data. What will be found is that the results have been inconclusive for defining fluent aphasic speech for a variety of reasons. The experimental procedures used by the researchers do not always allow for the problems of using fluent aphasic participants. For example, it is not always clear what comprehension problems the participants have and whether the presence of comprehension problems could account for some of the results. Obviously, if the subject has diminished comprehension, a defining feature of Wernicke's aphasia, then participation within an experiment is more problematic, and this factor may be part and parcel of the reason why these subjects perform differently from non-fluent or agrammatic subjects rather than a difference in linguistic representation. Secondly, fluent aphasic speakers very often have visual field defects. Even if these are fairly minor, they should be taken into account if experimental procedures require the subjects to respond to visual stimuli. In the absence of any reference to visual problems, the reader assumes that the subjects have normal vision, but it would be reassuring to have this information made explicit. Thirdly, whether or not visual field deficits coexist with the aphasia, most fluent aphasic speakers will have some type of acquired dyslexia and therefore this is a factor that should be taken into account if the experiment involves reading. Lastly, in this non-exhaustive list, there is the issue of individual variation. This factor applies equally to any group of aphasic speakers. What holds for a group does not necessarily hold for an individual with Wernicke's aphasia and the small numbers used by many researchers compounds the problem of generalising from the results gained.

There has been considerable debate in the literature about the validity of group studies and the assumptions that go with these studies. By and large, though, this debate has been confined to work in agrammatism although the same arguments hold for fluent aphasia. To some extent, the criticism is even more apt when applied to fluent aphasia. This is because there are more recognised syndromes subsumed under fluent aphasia, as outlined in chapter 1, and considerable variation. Whether or not, though, the variation between these syndromes is any greater than the variation that exists among patients diagnosed as having Broca's aphasia is not known. It is true that comprehension varies across fluent aphasic groups but it also does across individuals with Broca's aphasia. To some extent, the recognised differences within the various fluent aphasic syndromes is helpful as long as one checks to see what type of fluent aphasic subject is being referred to in any one study.

If studies are examined in their chronological order, then it can be seen how the explanations have developed over time. In some cases, explanations have become more sophisticated as more exact and subtle deficits are exposed. On the other hand, when we look at a range of studies that do not share the same theoretical interpretation of aphasic data, it is difficult to integrate the findings into a coherent explanation or even description of aphasia.

Summary

In this chapter we have examined in some detail studies that have claimed a syntactic explanation for language deficits in Broca's aphasia, or more often, agrammatism. However, while a syntactic deficit underlies both production and comprehension problems in agrammatic aphasia, the exact nature of the explanation is different for production and comprehension deficits. A central plank of this argument is that the nature of the production and comprehension deficits in agrammatism and the explanation of these deficits are exclusive to this condition. A number of on-line studies have produced what looks like supporting data, but we have also noted that there are experimental data that reveal that some fluent aphasic listeners may show a similar pattern of comprehension deficits to that claimed for agrammatism. In the next chapter we will look in more detail at comprehension problems in fluent aphasia.

6 *Comprehension and processing problems in fluent aphasia*

Introduction

Tests of comprehension give some insights into language abilities, highlighting the components of language that have been preserved, as well as those that are damaged. A different picture may emerge from that formed by looking solely at production data, but observed differences do not necessarily support the view that differences in performance indicate separate representation for input and output, as we have discussed in previous chapters. Differences may arise because of problems that compound the central language deficit. Problems at the phonological/phonetic level of representation can interfere with the pronunciation of words and thus we would not necessarily expect production and comprehension abilities to be parallel in all tasks. But, in the absence of pronunciation problems, we would expect problems with, for example, understanding certain syntactic structures or certain lexical items to be reflected in production tasks if there is a common central language module. In fact, to date, there is no convincing evidence that production and comprehension deficits do parallel one another, especially in agrammatic aphasia as we have discussed in chapter 5. Differences between production and comprehension abilities in aphasic speakers are taken as evidence that aphasia is a disorder of language processes rather than of language representation. But in fluent aphasia, production and comprehension of complex sentences are often compromised, suggesting that there is some parallelism in this type of aphasia.

In the previous chapter we reviewed a number of on-line studies where the performance in non-fluent and fluent aphasia has been compared, and now, in this chapter, the emphasis will be on off-line tasks and on comprehension abilities. Off-line tasks are used extensively in clinical practice and as far as the aphasic speaker and his/her conversational partners are concerned, it is off-line performance that is of paramount interest. Such tasks give an idea of how well the listener is able to understand language and which factors enhance, and which detract, from understanding. Even when on-line tasks do demonstrate superior processing performance, this is largely irrelevant to the person with aphasia. Part of coping with aphasia comes from a greater awareness of day-to-day abilities and developing strategies to deal with the changed language abilities. This is especially true for those with Wernicke's aphasia, for their families and for those with whom they have daily contact.

Comprehension loss and clinical presentation

The comprehension deficit in fluent aphasia, and especially in Wernicke's aphasia, is usually apparent without specialised testing. This contrasts with the comprehension deficit associated with two other fluent aphasias, conduction and anomic aphasia, and with non-fluent aphasia. Most patients within these diagnostic categories appear to understand spoken language and it is only by specific testing that a problem may be revealed. (Some classifications do not include comprehension deficits in these two syndromes.) In contrast to non-fluent aphasic speakers, Wernicke's speakers exhibit obvious, and sometimes florid, problems with comprehension. This apparent difference has, since the late nineteenth century, been a major diagnostic factor. However, as with all aphasic symptoms, the severity of the deficit in fluent aphasia varies considerably, both from patient to patient and individually, across tasks and over time. It is possible for the problems with comprehension to be moderate or mild, especially when there has been some improvement over time and problems can be masked. Some speakers with fluent aphasia and good interactional skills can hide their comprehension problems especially if the conversation is limited to social pleasantries (although this is unlikely to be under conscious control). In a brief meeting where exchanges are limited to social exchanges, the inexperienced listener may not detect that the aphasic speaker has comprehension problems. Family members may be puzzled by what they perceive to be the fluent aphasic speaker's reduced willingness to listen and to co-operate. For people involved with fluent aphasic people, explanation and demonstration of the difficulties experienced by the speaker with fluent aphasia can be very helpful for the family and may contribute to more harmonious conversations and time together.

A mild comprehension deficit may only be revealed by careful testing that not only decontextualises language but also separates meaning carried by lexical items and meaning that is dependent on syntax. Fluent aphasic listeners can experience more difficulties understanding sentences with complex syntax than sentences with simple syntactic structure, as we will see below. Once we start to investigate whether syntax contributes to the comprehension deficit in fluent aphasia, we see that features considered to be diagnostic of agrammatism may not be exclusive to that syndrome. It has been accepted for a long time that whereas lesions in the frontal lobe may be associated with syntactic difficulties, lesions in the temporal or temporal-parietal lobe are associated with semantic difficulties. Although this is broadly true, and preliminary brain studies tend to confirm this as a broad generalisation as we saw in chapter 1, a small but increasing number of studies show that there is not always such a stark difference.

Although a comprehension deficit nearly always presents problems both to the aphasic person and to conversational partners, the person with Wernicke's aphasia may be unaware that he has problems understanding language, especially in the early days immediately after the onset of aphasia, even when the comprehension problem is severe. Part of the rehabilitation process may involve the fluent aphasic speaker coming to realise that he/she is not always, or maybe hardly ever, comprehensible. This is a hard lesson and, when the revelation comes, the outcome may be that morale decreases as the aphasic speaker begins to understand the severity of his/her language disorder. On the other hand, lack of insight creates difficulties in day-to-day life and may have serious consequences. The person with aphasia may accuse others of not listening or of deliberately misunderstanding them. Patients may be unable to understand the explanations given to them by medical staff concerning their admission to hospital, for example, especially when there are no accompanying physical signs or when an initial hemiparesis rapidly improves. The improvement of a mild hemiparesis may be interpreted as a sign that all is well again despite a persisting severe aphasia. Patients may become agitated and angry. They may accuse staff or family of wrongdoing and of conspiring with the medical staff to keep them in hospital against their will. In severe cases, they may demand to be discharged, much to their family's distress. As hospital care changes in the UK, the possibility of extended stays becomes less likely and self-discharge is less likely to occur.

The language of the affected person may be so disturbed that neither hospital staff nor family understand what the patient is saying, and reasoned discussion is impossible. One patient of mine discharged himself from an acute ward, signing his own discharge papers as he left. He thought he was being detained in hospital for malign reasons and was being held against his will. As his aphasia improved, this elderly man with severe Wernicke's aphasia would complain to me that when he went out to his club or local bar, people would talk in a way he could not understand to exclude him deliberately. Not surprisingly, his wife found life very difficult. When volunteer visitors arrived at his house he assumed they were uninvited workmen and threw them out despite the pleadings of his wife and the attempted explanations of the two visitors.

Another patient, living in a large city, reported that he was misunderstood when, having locked himself out of his car, he tried to ask for help. He conveyed to me that this was because many people living in the town were foreigners and couldn't speak English. This was not the case. Why he was not understood was because a large part of his speech lacked meaning, known as jargon aphasia. (Jargon aphasia is a term used to describe speech that retains the sounds and intonation of the language but words are meaningless.) A stranger listening to him had not the advantage of knowing the speaker and may have never have come across a person with aphasia. The stranger would certainly not know about the speaker and would be limited, therefore, in guessing accurately what the aphasic speaker was trying to say. It is interesting to note that he wasn't able to use gesture effectively in this episode.

As his therapist, I was able to understand his story when he later related it to me. In a more relaxed and supportive situation, he was able to gesture, use facial expression and achieve a few salient single words. We also used a series of questions and answers, and my attempts at trying to understand his story were aided by my knowledge of his life and the supplementary explanations given by his wife. This particular man was an even-natured person, ever optimistic and ready to try new challenges. Even so, he had, if I had interpreted him correctly, arrived at not only an incorrect explanation for why he had not succeeded in securing help, but also a rather malevolent, gloomy one. It is easy to see how such patients may appear to be paranoid and how a differential diagnosis between this type of aphasia and psychiatric disturbances can be difficult. We have seen in chapter 2 that the behaviour disturbances that may accompany this lack of self-awareness can lead to problems of differential diagnosis.

Abstract concepts and two-dimensional diagrams: a historical perspective

Descriptions of the production deficits associated with aphasia have been around for centuries. Benton and Joynt (1960) offer a survey of historical descriptions that starts with the Hippocratic writings but they conclude that what they call 'sensory aphasia', known now as Wernicke's aphasia, was probably not recognised until Wernicke's description in his seminal monograph of 1874. (Not all aphasiologists have always agreed with this interpretation; see, for example, Benton 1964.) As we have seen in chapter 1, Wernicke was concerned with the notion of memory, concept formation and 'word concept'. He postulated that there were two stages in auditory comprehension. Firstly, a word as an auditory stimulus is transmitted via subcortical tracts to the sensory speech centre in the temporal lobe. This is the stage of 'primary identification': the word is perceived but not understood. The acoustic images then arouse the related concepts in what Wernicke referred to as the 'secondary identification' or 'word-meaning-comprehension' (Eggert 1977:36). Thus damage to the temporal lobe area would result in a sensory aphasia marked by poor auditory comprehension, a copious confused output, literal and verbal paraphasias, word-finding difficulties and problems with writing and reading (Eggert 1977:37). To the best of my knowledge, comprehension of sentences was not considered separately from comprehension of single words. In a wide-ranging paper, Head (1920:397) mentions Wernicke's work on the link between auditory comprehension and damage to the first left convolution. Head's ideas about aphasia were based on his experiences gained from examining patients with vascular lesions and then, following the First World War, young men 'struck down in the full pride of health', but his work did not lead to a clear description of comprehension problems either. What he describes as *semantic aphasia* includes a condition where 'the patient may understand each word or short phrase . . . but the ultimate meaning fails him' (p. 409). This finding would fit with the patient having access to lexical semantics but not being able to parse the syntax of the sentence in order to access meaning of that sentence. Notwithstanding Head's attack on Wernicke, Wernicke has had a lasting effect on how aphasia is viewed and, in many ways, new ideas are, in reality, ideas recycled from the nineteenth-century neuro-anatomist.

Although Wernicke's work was published more than one hundred years ago, his ideas about comprehension as a cognitive activity, involving at least two levels or stages, has endured and continues to influence models of language processing. Clinicians are familiar with patients who hear and repeat words but fail to recognise them as real words. When told, for example, that an object is a *clock*, a patient may respond by saying 'a clock, a clock, that doesn't sound right to me'. Or a common type of response is 'Clock? Clock? Well you could call it that but I don't'. By contrast, a patient might ask what something is called but, when told that the object in question is a clock, respond by saying 'a clock, a clock, no I don't know what that means'. In Wernicke's model, the first patient who cannot recognise that *clock* is a real word would have what he calls a deficit at the 'primary identification' stage. The patient in the second example, who cannot access the meaning of the word *clock*, has a deficit at Wernicke's 'secondary identification' stage. If a patient can neither recognise the word as a word nor associate the word with a correct meaning, then the deficit is, presumably, at both stages. It could be argued that such a patient need only have a deficit at the first, auditory, stage because if it's not recognised as a word, then, how can the listener access meaning? However, although deficits can be found which implicate both stages, it does not seem to be true that these stages are accessed serially. It is common for individuals with Wernicke's aphasia to perform poorly on tasks that investigate their ability to access auditory information (e.g. whether two words rhyme or share the same initial sounds) and yet to demonstrate understanding of the same words.

The first type of deficit resembles what would be categorised, under clinical models of language processing, as a deficit at the level of the auditory analyser or the phonological input buffer. Such deficits can be confirmed by tests such as judging between real and non-words. In the given example, the patient would not be able to judge reliably that *clock* was a real word. The second type of comprehension deficit is revealed when the patient is given a test of word meaning. There are various test protocols used. For example, the patient may be required to select a single picture from an array when given orally presented words; he may be asked if simple definitions match the target word; he may be required to indicate the correct definition for a series of single words. In the example given above, the patient would not be able to match the word *clock* to a picture or definition. Using the same kind of single-word processing model, this deficit would be assumed to be at the central semantic level, especially if both written and spoken input produced the same results.

Wernicke postulated that these different types of deficit, or stages of comprehension, arose from damage to different parts of the cortical and sub-cortical regions and that intact performance depended on an intact brain and the functioning of each part. Wernicke's diagram of auditory comprehension shows two stages, which are in part anatomical and in part abstract. The first stage, the word-sound identification stage involves subcortical tracts and the mes-sage/impulse leading to the sensory speech area. The second stage of word-meaning comprehension depicts cortical tracts leading to conceptualisation (Eggert 1977:39). Damage to the sensory area would, Wernicke claimed, lead to a sensory aphasia or what is now known as Wernicke's aphasia. This deficit, he noted, included a marked auditory deficit. Damage to the subcortical area would lead to what he called a subcortical sensory aphasia or word deafness (Eggert 1977:37).

It was diagrams such as this that led some critics to assume that the claim was for an isomorphic relationship between function and cortical area and to Henry Head's well-known attack on 'diagram makers'. He complained that diagram makers 'deduced (that) the mechanism of speech embodied it in a schematic form' and that from diagrams based on a priori assumptions they deduced defective functioning that must follow destruction of each 'centre or inter-nucleial path'. He claimed that the 'author(s) twisted the clinical facts to suit the lesions . . . deduced from his pet scheme' and said of these researchers that they were inclined to 'lop and twist the clinical facts to fit the Procrustean bed of the hypothetical conceptions' (Head 1920:306). It is, perhaps, not surprising, given the way the world works, that investigations into brain–language relationships swing between those based on a concept of integration of neural activity and those dedicated to the notion of a more precise relationship between function and cortical site. Following a search for a more integrated concept of cortical functioning, and how this impacts on our understanding of aphasia, many current studies are investigating the link between neural structure and language functioning. Once again the search is for localised sites that can be identified with elements of language processing (e.g. Hagoort, Brown and Osterhout 1999, Smith and Geva 2000). Caplan (2000) provides an excellent summary of the work in this field conducted by him and his colleagues.

Wernicke, while specifying the lesion site that was associated with sensory aphasia, also developed a model of functioning, constituting stages that were associated with cerebral sites and connections between those stages. It does not follow, though, that the process described by Wernicke was, necessarily, a serial process even though the existence of arrows between the stages of his diagram would suggest this. If the process of comprehension is a serial process in which each stage is essential, then presumably a deficit at the 'primary identification' stage would always be associated with a deficit at the 'secondary identification' stage. This is not always found in clinical practice. Indeed, Wernicke's work was based on the different types of language disturbances he was observing in his medical practice and, from the case studies that he published, there is no evidence that he set about looking for clear evidence of these different stages, or at least did not give them as illustrations. But it is clear that he did assume that there was a relationship between type of language disorder and site of lesion although his concept of the process embraced psychological processes as well as neurological ones.

Over one hundred years later, his notions of stages and levels, although given different terminology, are still abroad, especially in clinical assessment. In a simple form, the PALPA assessment that we considered in chapter 3 examines word-finding difficulties using some similar concepts. In the model of language processing used by these authors, there is no attempt to correlate function to site of lesion, as Wernicke did, but there is the same attempt to break down the process of understanding language, or at least understanding single words, into stages of mental activity. The stages are auditory discrimination, where individual phonemes can be recognised; word recognition, where a real word can be distinguished from a non-word; a semantic stage, where meaning of the word is accessed. Intact auditory discrimination allows one to repeat real and non-words as well as real words without accessing meaning of that word. Outside the phonetic class, the ability to repeat non-words is necessary when hearing a new proper noun such as a surname, place name, street name and so on, or a foreign word. The ability to reject non-words permits non-aphasic speakers to reject mispronunciations, and the ability to connect word form with meaning allows us to understand what we hear.

Components of comprehension

Although it is usually a fairly straightforward matter to identify the presence of a comprehension deficit by means of conversation or some simple tests, it is much less straightforward to understand the nature of the deficit. Which components of language make understanding difficult for the aphasic listener? For more than a hundred years it has been accepted that listeners with Wernicke's aphasia have problems with word meaning. Some examples have been given above and, as we have seen, investigations and especially clinical investigations of comprehension in aphasia put great emphasis on the understanding of single words. Clinical investigation of single-word comprehension focuses largely on the understanding of concrete picturable nouns. It is only comparatively recently that materials for testing the understanding of verbs have been available. It is clear that problems of associating meaning with word form will interfere with understanding language but grammar, too, plays a part in understanding language.

Non-linguistic factors in comprehension

Although the data supporting the claim about the types of sentences that agrammatic listeners find difficult are robust, there is no universal agreement why this might be. There could be non-linguistic explanations of why passives, object-relative sentences and so on might be more difficult for these patients. The sentences that cause difficulty are non-canonical, less frequent and longer than active sentences. The cause might not be the grammar per se of these sentences but other, non-linguistic, factors. Length of sentence might interact with a reduced auditory memory that often accompanies aphasia, while the frequency and canonicity factors could militate against ease of processing.

Psycholinguistic research has shown that these factors are related to speed of lexical and sentential processing for non-aphasic speakers as well as aphasic listeners. To date, there is no consensus on whether errors in comprehension are caused by a disruption of central representation, within the mental lexicon and/or the grammar, or by disrupted access to these domains, or a concomitant cognitive problem subsequent to brain damage but separate from aphasia.

In a number of papers during the last fifteen years or so (e.g. Just and Carpenter 1992, Miyake, Carpenter and Just 1994), it has been argued that errors of comprehension could be accounted for by restrictions in working memory. This is on the basis that both normal and aphasic subjects show increased reaction time as sentence complexity is increased (Miyake, Carpenter and Just 1994). Reduction in short-time memory is often a further consequence of the brain damage that caused the aphasia. Could it be, then, that difficulty in understanding connected speech arises because of the limitations in short-term memory? The more complex the sentence, the longer it is likely to be and the more difficult to understand, but short-term memory, that is a general rather than a language specific cognitive process, is not necessarily the culprit. There is an increasing consensus that problems with parsing sentences is separate from any limitation in a phonological STM deficit (Inglis 2003). Other groups of researchers formulate the relationship between STM and parsing rather differently.

Martin and her group of colleagues claim that deficits in verbal short-term memory and lexical processing share a common underlying deficit (Martin and Gupta 2004:214). Reviewing a large body of work from their own and other laboratories, they note that there is evidence that properties of the language system impact on performances in short-term memory tasks which 'suggest that the relationship between lexical processing and verbal short-term memory is bidirectional'. They take a model of lexical processing in which activation, maintenance and decay of phonological and semantic representations and connections account for memory restrictions, primacy and recency effects as well as phonological and semantic errors. The interactive activation of the lexical system maintains information within that system and is 'a form of short-term memory' (p. 225). Thus the understanding and production of words depends on the integrity of those activation systems. When severely disrupted, understanding or production of a single word may be affected. When the disruption is mild, the system may be able to process single but not multiple words. Thus they claim that all individuals with aphasia should also present with verbal STM deficits although not all individuals with STM deficits will have obvious aphasic symptoms (p. 225).

While the data from repetition tasks involving words and non-words provide insights into the mechanism of word processing, it is difficult to integrate these findings with those that investigate the effect of word class or with results from studies of sentence processing. Presumably, the processing component of single words can be affected by the syntactic component. As we will see below, people with aphasia may have good comprehension of single words, that is, their processing seems to be functioning efficiently, but, given the same words in a syntactically complex sentence, comprehension is diminished.

Hagoort, Brown and Osterhout (1999) give a summary of some of the issues involved in processing sentences. They describe the process of 'structure building' as one in which lexical items, or lemmas, are accessed and incrementally grouped to form syntactic structures. The authors describe a process of on-line parsing that could be used on hearing a sentence. The whole sentence structure is not retrieved from memory but built up incrementally, as it is in production. Components of the sentence may not be immediately assigned within the sentence structure but need to be 'kept active', especially in the sentence types discussed above, until the syntactic structure is completed. By 'keeping alive' there is an assumption that components are held in working memory until the complete sentence can be parsed. The length of storage and/or amount of processing involved will vary with the complexity of the sentence. The computational resources required for parsing a simple active sentence are assumed to be less than those required for more complex sentences. The more complex the sentence, the more computational resources required. However, definitions of 'complexity' vary. There are claims that the number of verbs, the number of propositions, the frequency of the sentence type all contribute to the varying demands on processing resources. Other strong claims are made about the contribution of syntactic structure, where the presence of moved constituents and co-indexing over short or long distances are complexity factors. Further, discourse factors, whether the sentence is 'discourse related', may be yet another candidate (Hickok and Avrutin 1995, 1996, Avrutin 2000). Hagoort and colleagues note that there is increasing evidence that syntactic, semantic and pragmatic information all play a role in determining the meaning of a sentence. Thus sentences given in a test situation where no additional contextual information is available may be understood less well than the same sentence within a communicative context where additional syntactic, semantic and pragmatic information is available. This view is widely held by clinicians.

So, there are at least four ways of explaining comprehension problems. A language deficit may arise from damage to a domain or domains of language. In this case, the aphasic listener would not have complete access to lexical meaning or meaning of certain sentences because of lexical or syntactic loss. It is hard to maintain a case for damage to central representation per se if this is conceived as deletion of operations or knowledge. In aphasia, written and spoken language can be affected differently as can output and input capacities. Performance on on-line and off-line tasks may differ. Comprehension can be aided by various cues and performance and can vary within one subject and across tasks. For example, an individual with aphasia may perform badly on sentence-comprehension tasks but well on judgement tasks where the same structures are used. Except in the most severe cases, we look for trends in the data: results are rarely categorical.

A second explanation may be that the grammar and lexicon are intact but access to either or both, or to part of either or both, is deficient. Thirdly, and closely related to the second explanation, grammar and the lexicon may stay intact but certain language-dedicated processing abilities may be at fault, as Zurif and colleagues claim. Here it is not just access but various language-dedicated processes, as yet underspecified, that are deficient. However, how dedicated language processes differ from grammatical operations is not made clear. Is a dedicated language processor the same as grammatical operations, and if not, how do they differ? The processor, if dedicated to language, must be constrained by grammatical rules, that is, the operations of the grammar. The data to date suggest that comprehension deficits arise from processing limitations, processing that is dedicated to language and thus involves syntactic and other linguistic constraints.

And finally, it could be that language deficits arise as a consequence of deficient general processing abilities that are, in turn, the consequence of brain damage. Working memory involved in processing can, it must follow, be seen as part of the general cognitive activity that impacts on the dedicated processing, or, as part of the dedicated process. This processing may in turn have separate components dedicated to separate language operations. Hagoort and colleagues (e.g. Hagoort and Kutas 1995, Hagoort Brown and Osterhout 1999) suggest that current information, gained from a whole range of experimental studies, points to the involvement of a number of specialised operations. One (or more) of these involves memory for long-distant structural relations, as in passive sentences, certain wh-questions and relative clauses. Such operations can be conceived, it would appear, as part of the grammar, the operational part of language. As such, it can be independently impaired following brain damage, as in agrammatism.

Reduced working memory capacity (RWMC) is found in people with fluent aphasia. It can be demonstrated in tasks such as word and digit recall and in sentence-comprehension tasks involving sentences with increasing complexity. If working memory could account for the sentence comprehension problems of agrammatic listeners, then we might predict that we would find the same pattern in fluent aphasia. If, however, the (grammatical) operations involved are associated with a specific region of the brain, say Broca's area, as Grodzinsky claims, then we would not expect to find similar deficits in aphasias that arise from temporal rather than from frontal lobe lesions. There are a number of studies that support this prediction of differential deficits. For example, a number of studies have used reaction times in psycholinguistic tasks: some of these we have looked at in the previous chapter. It has been found that aphasic performance depends on (a) the type of aphasia of the subject and (b) sentence type (Swinney, Zurif and Nicol 1989, Shapiro and Levine 1990, Shapiro, Gordon, Hack and Killackey 1993). Martin (1995) reviews other data as evidence against the RWMC hypothesis. Among the studies she reviews she considers that a study by Blumstein, Katz, Goodglass, Shrier and Dworsky (1985) is one that could be used in support of a RWMC hypothesis, although only for Wernicke's aphasia. These researchers found that increasing pauses at syntactic boundaries did improve comprehension for the Wernicke's group although not for conduction aphasics. Pausing did not improve the comprehension for global aphasics or Broca's aphasics. However, although the comprehension of Wernicke's subjects improved with increased pauses, this improvement did not relate to sentence complexity. If complex sentences are difficult because of RWMC and if pausing assists working memory, then we would expect to see an interaction.

Understanding words and sentences

It is reasonable, then, to assume that comprehension deficits arise from a number of interacting factors. Many fluent aphasics have RWMC but other linguistic factors contribute to their comprehension difficulties. These factors are both lexical and syntactic and involve processing that is constrained by grammatical rules and operations. The lexical features of the comprehension deficit are the most obvious. Fluent aphasic subjects have problems with associating word form with meaning and problems with other assumed stages or levels in the process of comprehending language. At a basic level, it can be demonstrated that fluent aphasic listeners have difficulty distinguishing between single phonemes. They find it difficult to judge whether or not words sound the same, whether they start with the same phoneme, and some have difficulty making rhyming judgements. They also, quite obviously, have difficulty with word meaning.

In Wernicke's aphasia, Benson notes, comprehension difficulties may be of different types. There may be difficulty with recognising and distinguishing between speech sounds and difficulty with relating what is heard to linguistic knowledge. He also quotes Lesser (1978) who talked about an inability 'to appreciate concepts' and a difficulty with 'mental manipulation of language'. Lesser (1978:148) also observes the difficulty in trying to isolate syntactic and semantic levels of difficulties in these patients.

Factors of frequency and length exert an influence but also the factor of word class and, within that, the lexical information that each word has. So, verbs may be more difficult for aphasic speakers to access than nouns because of the semantic and syntactic information held, and within the class of verbs, type of verb may be associated with greater or lesser ease of access. Verbs vary in the number of complements they permit and the types of phrasal structures the complements can take. For example, *to eat* and *to devour* have similar meanings but take a different number of arguments. Both need an *agent* but only *devour* takes an obligatory theme: *he eats* but **he devours*. This variation impacts on aphasic speakers, especially those with Broca's aphasia rather than Wernicke's and especially in production tasks (Zingeser and Berndt 1990, Damasio and Tranel 1993).

Dissociations found across aphasia types that arise from damage to different cortical areas strengthen both the concepts of the modular nature of language and the localisation view of aphasia. Different components of language have different cortical representations. Thus lexical semantic deficits may dissociate from deficits that are syntactic in nature. The Broca's subjects in the Zurif experiments were thought to have difficulties not with syntactic representation per se but with processing grammatical relations. In contrast, the Wernicke's subjects were shown to have intact access to trace. Their semantic problems were thought to underlie the lack of pattern in their reaction times to the verbs with varying numbers of potential arguments.

But while we may wish to keep the notion of two sorts of comprehension problems separate, we can still hold that both types of impairment can be manifested in the same type of aphasia. Increasingly, there are findings that suggest that lexical and syntactic deficits of comprehension cannot be divided neatly between the two canonical aphasia types. In particular, there is some evidence that, in addition to problems in distinguishing between speech sounds and with understanding words, some fluent aphasic speakers also have the same difficulties in understanding the same types of sentence structures that agrammatic speakers have.

Comprehension difficulties with sentences

The comprehension of certain sentence structures by some agrammatic subjects has led to considerable research activity. A veritable industry sprang up during the last two decades of the twentieth century and the debate continues. The excitement started when, contrary to expectations, it was found that patients with seemingly good comprehension for conversational speech were unable to demonstrate sentence comprehension of certain sentence types. Caramazza and Zurif (1976) found that patients who were diagnosed as having Broca's aphasia and conduction aphasia failed to understand sentences containing centrally embedded relative clauses if the NPs of the sentence were reversible, that is when either NP could, plausibly, be the agent of the sentence. So, given the sentence *the lion that the tiger is chasing is fat* they would be unable to identify which of the NPs was the agent and which was the patient. Using a picture-selection task, two types of distractors were offered: lexical distractors showing either an alternative verb or adjective and distractors showing the reversal of the agent and patient/theme. The findings were important as they clearly demonstrated that Broca's patients did have problems with comprehension and, furthermore, problems with understanding were a function of sentence type. This finding fuelled the view that Broca's aphasia involved a syntactic deficit. Unfortunately, the conduction aphasic subjects also showed this pattern.

However, the conclusion that the errors in picture selection arose from a syntactic deficit may not be well grounded. It may be that the results indicate that comprehension was dependent on accessing not only lexical, but also semantic, information, and the need for both types of information caused the difficulties. Errors involved both types of distractors. The lexical and the thematic role reversals were chosen. Thus it is not possible to say why the subjects failed the tasks, but their incorrect responses suggest that lexical and syntactic processes were faulty. As Martin and Blossom-Stach (1986:201) noted, the subjects could have been showing both syntactic and semantic deficits. The Caramazza and Zurif (1976) findings have often been taken as evidence that Broca's, not Wernicke's, aphasia involves problems with syntactic parsing. In fact their claim was more modest and they were cautious about their claims for Wernicke's aphasia. There have been a number of subsequent studies that suggest that at least some individuals with Wernicke's aphasia may have problems parsing certain sentence types.

Martin and Blossom-Stach presented a case study of one Wernicke's aphasic subject. They examined his understanding of a set of active and passive sentences and found that the subject's performance varied according to the type of distractors used. When given lexical distractors, either alternative NPs or verbs, the subject performed well on both active and passive sentences. When given reverse roles as distractors, the subject's performance fell for both active and passive sentences. The subject scored 65 per cent correct for all sentences when given reverse role distractors compared to 95 per cent correct when given lexical distractors. The authors concluded that the poor performance on the reversal picture pairs in the comprehension tasks suggested that the errors in comprehension did not depend on semantic processing but implicated the subject's processing of the syntactic information in sentences. They concluded that their subject's 'deficiencies in production and comprehension were due to syntactic impairments' (p. 229). Similar findings have been reported elsewhere as we will now consider.

Comprehension on single verbs and sentences

Even if fluent aphasia comprehension deficits do not have an underlying syntactic problem, it is becoming clear that (some) fluent aphasic people find complex sentences more difficult to understand than simple canonical sentences. In studies by Caplan, Waters and Hilderbrandt (1997) and Balogh and Grodzinsky (2000) fluent aphasic subjects had a similar performance to that of agrammatic subjects on a sentence-comprehension task. Recently, Bastiaanse and Edwards (2000, 2004) have reported on comprehension abilities in four groups of aphasic patients, English-speaking Broca's and Wernicke's patients and Dutch-speaking Broca's and Wernicke's patients. They found that both Wernicke's as well as Broca's subjects had significantly more difficulty with understanding sentences that had a non-canonical structure. All four groups understood the actives and subject-cleft sentences significantly better than the passive and object-cleft sentences.

In this next section of this chapter we will look at some similar data. There is some overlap between the subjects reported here and those in the Bastiaanse and Edwards' papers (henceforth B and E). The group we discuss here comprises English-speaking fluent aphasic subjects, some of whom were included in the B and E studies. The fluent subjects in the B and E studies were all diagnosed as Wernicke's. Here the group of fluent aphasic subjects has been extended to include some subjects with anomic aphasia, but despite this, the results are very similar. All the subjects were tested with a series of tests from the Verb and Sentence Test (Bastiaanse, Edwards and Rispens 2002). This comprises a series of tests that examine verb and sentence production and comprehension and has been described in chapter 3. In table 6.1 the scores for two of these tests

Table 6.1 *VAST scores for verb and sentence comprehension for 12 fluent aphasic patients*

Subject	Gender	Age	Years education	Diagnosis	Time since onset (months)	Verb comp (40 items)	Sentence comp (40 items)
JoH	M	76	12	CVA Wernicke's	63	34	20
MG	M	65	15	CVA Wernicke's	103	38	24
MF	F	81	12	CVA Wernicke's	15	28	20
IM	M	70	8	CVA Wernicke's	7	37	22
MB	F	75	9	CVA Wernicke's	6	33	27
EH	F	70	12	CVA Wernicke's	3	36	30
JS	M	60	12	CVA Wernicke's	6	37	24
MS	F	60	12	CVA mild Wernicke's	15	40	33
DC	M	56	15	CVA mild Wernicke's	9	33	35
DM	M	72	12	CVA anomic	12	37	38
CG	M	58	12	CVA anomic	20	39	38
TR	M	70	15	CVA anomic	17	37	39

Mean for Verb Comprehension test for 9 Wernicke's subjects = 35.1; range = 28–40
Mean for Verb Comprehension test for all 12 fluent subjects = 36.2; range = 28–40
Mean for Sentence Comprehension test for 9 Wernicke's subjects = 26.1; range = 20–30
Mean for Sentence Comprehension test for all 12 fluent subjects = 29.2; range = 20–39
Mean for Verb Comprehension test for 22 controls = 39.7; range = 38–40
Mean for Sentence Comprehension test for 22 controls = 39.9; range = 39–40

are displayed with the subjects' details. Some preliminary data have already been discussed in chapter 3. Here we will consider the results from two tests of comprehension in more detail.

Aphasia type for each subject was decided by results on the BDAE, clinical tests and spontaneous speech samples. Three of the twelve fluent aphasic subjects were thought to have anomic aphasia, as their comprehension was judged by their clinicians to be only slightly impaired but they had considerable problems in producing words, especially nouns, in spontaneous speech and confrontational naming tasks. In fact, as we have seen in chapter 3, all but one of these subjects also had problems accessing verbs as single words. The exception was TR, who had made a good recovery and whose comprehension at the time of testing was virtually at ceiling. TR also had the highest score for producing verbs as single words. We can see that the scores for both the Verb Comprehension tests and the Sentence Comprehension test confirm that these three anomic subjects are better comprehenders than those in the Wernicke's group. All three subjects had improved since the time of onset of aphasia and had originally presented as moderate or mild Wernicke's aphasics in early period post-onset of the aphasia.

Results from the two sub-tests shown in table 6.1 repeat some of the data given earlier, but we will now examine the results in more detail. The two tests we will now consider probe the comprehension of verbs as single words and the comprehension of four sentence types (actives, passive, subject and object clefts). Test procedures include word– and sentence–picture matching tasks. These scores show very clearly the difference in comprehension between the anomic group (the last three on the table) and those with Wernicke's aphasia. Looking at the scores for the single verbs first, we can see that all the subjects have mild to moderate loss for verbs as single words: one (CG) of the anomic group fell within the normal range. Looking at the performance of the Wernicke's group, we can see that eight of the nine subjects performed less well on the sentence-comprehension task than on the task of selecting pictures representing single verbs. Most of the subjects were better at understanding verbs as single words than they were at understanding the sentences used in this test. However, one subject, DC had the reverse picture, performing less well on the single-verb task than he did on the sentence-comprehension task. In fact, he achieved the highest score for sentence comprehension of the Wernicke's group but the second lowest score for the verb test.

Subjects in the anomic group are so near ceiling that the difference between the two tasks, verb comprehension and sentence comprehension, is small. None of them, however, actually reached ceiling. They all had some discernible residual comprehension deficit, albeit small. Patients with similar mild residual

Table 6.2 *Wernicke's comprehension of four sentence types: % correct*

Subject	Active	Subject Cleft	Passive	Object cleft	Total % correct
JoH	60	70	50	30	50
MG	50	70	50	70	60
MF	50	50	30	60	40
IM	60	80	30	50	55
MB	80	60	80	60	67
EH	90	80	60	70	75
JS	80	80	40	40	60
MS	80	100	80	70	82
DC	100	100	80	70	87
MEANS	72	77	55.5	57.7	

problems often complain that they have difficulty following conversations and television programmes and have to change their reading materials. This test has revealed something of these difficulties. After all, if a listener fails to compre- hend one or two sentences in forty, then this could have serious consequences for following conversations or dialogue. People with mild aphasia may be perform- ing near ceiling on experimental tests but still show problems in everyday life (McCann and Edwards 2003). Correct scores may be achieved at the expense of speed. It has been shown that treatment can change accuracy or speed. Edwards, Tucker and McCann (2004) reported on a patient with mild aphasia whose scores and verb tests improved marginally but improved significantly on speed of response.

Comprehending sentences

Why should these subjects show greater difficulty in understanding sentences than they do in understanding single words if syntax is intact? Earlier in the chap- ter we briefly considered the influence of working memory on comprehension abilities. As we look further into these results we will see that working-memory deficits, even if present in these subjects, cannot, by themselves, account for the results. We can see in table 6.2 that, as a group, those with Wernicke's aphasia are better at the canonical sentences, the active and subject clefts than with the non-canonical, the passives and object clefts. As a group of fluent aphasic lis- teners, they perform better on actives and subject-cleft sentences where there is a canonical order of thematic roles than they do on passives and object-cleft sen- tences where the order is non-canonical. The difference between the canonical and non-canonical sentences is significant. Seven of the subjects scored higher on the canonical compared with the non-canonical sentences (JoH, MF, IM, EH, JS, MS and DC). Two of the subjects, MG and MB, were equally poor on canonical and non-canonical. However, although there is a difference in scores between the canonical and non-canonical sentences, only four of the subjects approach the above chance for canonical and at chance performance for non-canonical pattern reported for Broca's aphasia: (JoH, MF, IM, JS). Here, chance is taken to be 45–55 per cent. Although the task was to select one of four pictures to match the sentence that was heard, errors overwhelmingly involved reverse roles. Over 80 per cent of all errors involved reverse role errors. Thus subjects were choosing between two, rather than four, possibilities. Further details are given in Bastiaanse and Edwards (2001).

If we look at these subjects as a group, the pattern of performance of these fluent aphasic speakers mimics that reported for agrammatic patients. As a group, these Wernicke's subjects are performing above chance for active and subject-cleft sentences but at chance for the passives and the object clefts: 70+ for canonical and 50+ for non-canonical as shown in table 6.2. These results are at odds with the strong claims that the pattern of sentence comprehension for fluent aphasic individuals differs from that found in agrammatism. Could it be that, although the overall pattern of sentence comprehension in these subjects looks very similar to that found in agrammatism, the cause of the errors is different? We have already noted in chapter 5 that patients with fluent aphasia can show the same pattern in sentence comprehension as agrammatic patients (Balogh and Grodzinsky 2000), but these authors claim that similar results do not necessarily arise from the same underlying disorder. We can make some deductions about the nature of the underlying nature of the disorder by looking at the types of errors produced. The nature of the errors made by the fluent aphasic subjects should, if the underlying disorder is different, differ from those made by agrammatic patients.

In this test there are three types of distractor picture.

1. Reverse role: a picture showing the same actors but in reverse agent/theme position. An example of a reverse-role picture where the target is *the woman rescues the man* would be one where the man is rescuing the woman.
2. Lexical: a picture where the agent/theme roles remain as in the target sentence but showing a different action. An example of a lexical distractor for the target *the woman rescues the man* would be a picture showing the woman hugging the man.

Table 6.3 *Number and % of role reversal, lexical and role reversal + lexical errors for twelve fluent aphasic subjects on the Sentence Comprehension test*

	Active		Subject cleft		Passive		Object cleft		Total	
Reverse role	22	85%	16	70%	38	95%	35	87%	111	86%
Lexical	2	7.6%	5	22%	1	1%	1	2.5%	9	7%
RR + lexical	2	7.6%	2	4.7%	1	1%	4	1%	9	7%
Total	26	20%	23	18%	40	31%	40	31%	129	

3. Reverse role + lexical distractor: combines the above. So for the target we are using, *the woman rescues the man,* the picture would show the man kissing the woman.

If errors involve lexical distractors, it would suggest that the problems with understanding arise from a difficulty in understanding the meaning of individual verbs. A choice of a target that depicts the same NPs but with reverse thematic roles, on the other hand, suggests that the listener is not able to use the syntax of the sentence to assign thematic role and thus arrive at the correct meaning. We can look at error type that this set of patients made in table 6.3. Percentages have been used despite the low values of the raw scores, to illustrate the large difference between error types when seen as a proportion of the types of errors made. It can be seen that, overwhelmingly, these fluent aphasic subjects made reverse-role errors on all sentence types. Although they made more errors in the passive and object-cleft sentences than they did on the active and subject-cleft sentences, the proportion of reverse-role errors for each sentence type is very high. Out of 129 errors, 111 (86 per cent) were reverse-role errors. This pattern held for all subjects (table 6.3) and for the nine Wernicke's subjects (table 6.4). A number of conclusions can be draw from these results. First, these findings are in line with what we would expect to find in fluent aphasia, including the different degrees of severity. Secondly, results demonstrate that understanding of language depends on the nature of the input; single words, in this case single verbs, were easier to understand, for most subjects, than were sentences. Thirdly, sentence structure impacts upon comprehension, and those sentences that are more complex in some way – for example, by not having canonical order of thematic roles – are more difficult to understand. More errors were found in the non-canonical sentences. Finally, the nature of the errors made by these subjects showed, overwhelmingly, that given a choice of distractors, the

Table 6.4 *Distribution of errors for 9 Wernicke's aphasic subjects: raw scores and percentages*

	Active		Subject cleft		Passive		Object cleft		Total of all errors	
Reverse role	21	84%	16	73%	38	95%	33	89%	108	86.4%
Lexical	2	8%	4	18%	1	2.5%	1	2.5%	8	6.4%
RR + lexical	2	8%	2	9%	1	2.5%	4	10%	9	7.2%
TOTAL	25	20%	22	17.6%	40	32%	38	30.4%	125	

errors were not random. All these subjects, irrespective of the level of deficit, made errors involving theta-role assignment. We need to consider the combined influence of the type of sentence and the implication of the type of error made.

It is clear that these subjects find the active and subject-cleft sentences significantly easier than passive and object-cleft sentences. Secondly, although reverse-role errors predominate in all sentence types, the proportions of reverse-role errors were higher for the passive and object-cleft sentences than for the active and subject-cleft sentences. The difference in the number of errors made in sentences with canonical theta-role order was significantly lower than the errors made in those sentences where there was a non-canonical theta-role order. Furthermore, the non-canonical sentences all involve moved sentence constituents, as discussed in the previous chapter. Thus, these subjects with fluent aphasia exhibited the same kind of pattern of sentence-comprehension deficit as that reported for agrammatic subjects. The distractors chosen in error point to problems in theta-role assignment exacerbated by sentence complexity. There is one important difference, however. The pattern of chance performance on non-canonical sentences and above-chance performance on the canonical sentences is found for the group but not for every member of the group. How can these results be interpreted? Do these patients have difficulty with assigning theta-roles and, if so, why doesn't chance performance result?

The ability to understand who the agent of an action is and who the recipient is is pretty fundamental. It can be conceived as a problem with parsing the syntactic structure or as a stage between syntactic and semantic representation. In these data, the listeners were less reliable at assigning thematic agent roles or 'mapping' between syntactic and semantic representation in the non-canonical sentences than they were in the canonical. It has been argued that difficulties exhibited by agrammatic subjects with these types of sentences indicate a problem with grammar. Do the results lead us to the same conclusion?

Theories differ in detail but a number involve trace and co-indexing. We have seen that Grodzinsky claims that trace is lost, while others, for example, Beretta (2001), suggest that the difference between these two types of sentences is not the presence of trace, but the presence of two dependencies in passives and object-cleft sentences and one in actives and subject clefts. If the co-indexing constraint is removed or damaged, then the aphasic listener will respond at chance level. Only some of our fluent aphasic subjects performed at chance on the non-canonical sentences, but seven of the nine found the non-canonical sentences more difficult to understand than the canonical.

The on-line trial we reviewed earlier by Sweeney and his colleagues showed that the Broca's but not the fluent aphasic subjects had problems with trace. These findings were not replicated by Blumstein and her colleagues, and recent work shows increasing evidence that subjects with fluent aphasia may have very similar comprehension profiles to those found in agrammatism. Our findings are in line with these and more recent findings of Luzzatti and his colleagues.

Luzzatti and his colleagues (2001) investigated sentence comprehension in Italian aphasics. They had eleven agrammatic subjects and sixteen fluent subjects, of whom six were conduction aphasics and ten were Wernicke's. They found that movement, in their study of a clitic object, influenced the performance of conduction and Wernicke's subjects as well as that of the agrammatic subjects. Like other researchers, they failed to show that there was a difference between the patterns of comprehension deficit in subjects with anterior lesions compared with subjects with posterior lesions. As a group, their fluent aphasic subjects performed less well than the agrammatic subjects and they concluded that if trace is implicated in agrammatism, then it must be implicated in fluent aphasia too. In their study, the comprehension deficit observed in the agrammatic subjects also occurred in the fluent aphasic subjects, but the deficit was more severe. The subjects I am reporting on are not generally more impaired in comprehension. What we have reported is the same kind of pattern that is found in agrammatism but with *higher* performance on non-canonical sentences and *lower* performance on canonical sentences than we find for the Broca's group. The scores converge.

Our findings also support the claims of Crain, Ni and Shankweiler (2001) that the pattern of sentence comprehension found in agrammatism can be replicated in other populations. Crain, Ni and Shankweiler refer to data from fluent aphasia but the report they cite is one covering an examination of one

Serbo-Croatian speaker. The data reported here, however, back their claims. Here we have found that not only does the pattern of sentence comprehension impairment found in speakers with fluent aphasia resemble that found in agrammatism but the fluent aphasic speakers also make the same types of errors. These errors point to a difficulty with assigning theta roles. Luzzatti and colleagues suggest that their results point to the existence of lexical damage to the thematic grid and/or assignment of the thematic roles. The errors made on the sentence-comprehension test we considered earlier in the chapter support this notion. However, on a different task, the performance of the same Wernicke's subjects suggested that access to lexical information about thematic roles may be dependant, at least to some degree, on the types of tasks given to subjects.

Verb arguments and thematic roles

If subjects have difficulty assigning thematic roles, then this should be visible in other types of tasks. One such task is a sentence-judgement task. The task we used was from the VAST. In this task, subjects listen to a series of forty sentences and judge whether the sentence is a 'good' sentence or a 'bad' sentence. An example of a 'good' sentence would be *the boy cooks the egg* and an example of a 'bad' sentence would be *the egg cooks the boy*. Half the sentences in this test have NPs that are semantically anomalous with the theta role required: half are well-formed sentences. The semantically anomalous sentences are all formed by using a NP which, semantically, can not function as Agent in the sentence. Four sentence types were used: actives, subject clefts, passives and object clefts. If subjects have difficulty assigning thematic roles, then this test should present difficulties for them. If they are able to make correct judgements, then information about thematic roles of NPs must be available at some level of representation. What was found was that, on the whole, subjects performed better on this test than their scores on the sentence-comprehension task predicted. Once again, though, errors were more common in the non-canonical sentences.

Subjects were given several examples to establish that they understood the procedure. The results are shown in table 6.5. Percentage correct for each subject is shown for the sentence-judgement task. Percentage correct is also shown for the two tests we considered earlier in the chapter, the verb-comprehension and the sentence-comprehension tests. We can thus make comparisons across three types of comprehension tasks. Five of the subjects conformed to the pattern of gaining the highest score for verb comprehension followed by sentence judgement, followed by sentence comprehension. A further two subjects

Table 6.5 *Percentage correct on verb-comprehension, sentence-judgement task and sentence-comprehension task:*
forty items in each test

Subject	Verb comprehension	Thematic role judgement	Sentence comprehension
JoH	85	80	50
MG	95	70	60
MF	70	82	50
IM	92	42	55
MB	82	75	67
EH	90	97	92
JS	92	67	60
MS	100	95	82
DC	82	48	87

(MF and EH) also found sentence comprehension more difficult than thematic role judgement but, unlike the majority of the group, gained a higher score on the judgement task than on the verb-comprehension task. Only two subjects were better on sentence comprehension than sentence judgement (IM and DC). The subject IM scored around chance on both tasks involving sentences, results that are in contrast with his score on the verb test. These scores suggest that IM has problems with sentence processing. He made eighteen errors in the sentence-comprehension task (22/40 items correct) of which sixteen were reverse errors. That is, he chose the distractor picture where the NP which had the role of theme in the target sentence was shown as agent. Given that he had difficulty with selecting pictures depicting the correct thematic role, it is not surprising that he found it difficult to judge correctly whether sentences had NPs in plausible thematic roles. Both of his scores on the tasks involving sentences are lower than his score for the single-verb test.

The scores of DC are more problematic. He scores above 80 per cent on both the single-verb test and the sentence-comprehension test but only at chance level on the judgement task. It could be that he has difficulty deciding on the acceptability of NPs as arguments within a sentence, but if that is the case, we would expect him to have problems with the non-canonical sentences in the sentence comprehension task. Although he was a relatively high scorer (35/40), all his errors involved the reverse-role distractor. This shows that his understanding of thematic roles of verb arguments is not secure. This fragility was exposed in the judgement task. This task involved auditory stimuli only, whereas the other two tasks where he gained higher scores had visual stimuli. This might have had an effect on this particular subject although there is no evidence that the mode of stimuli affected the other subjects. We will now turn to verb arguments.

The results of the VAST test that we have spent some time considering confirm that a comprehension deficit is more than loss of meaning of words in Wernicke's aphasia. The results of the sentence-comprehension tests suggest that syntactic structure and canonical order of thematic roles, that is, order of verb arguments, plays an important part. Studies have shown that Wernicke's subjects, unlike Broca's subjects, do not have access to all the arguments of a verb, at least when tested on-line. In the test results we have reviewed, the subjects had good understanding of verbs when heard as single words. They were able to select between distractors that depicted actions and those that depicted objects. However, this knowledge was not sufficient to give them reliable access to the meaning of passive and object-cleft sentences. Furthermore, when given two sentences that showed NPs in reverse positions, they consistently failed to choose the correct target in this test.

Watching many of these subjects performing these tests, one is struck by their indecision when they reach non-canonical sentences. Some of the subjects shake their heads when confronted with the passive and object cleft sentences and gesture that they won't be able to do the sentence. They point from one picture to the other trying to choose between the reverse roles. Once a target is selected, they may look quizzically at the examiner and, on completion of the test, ask to go back to the items they knew they had difficulty with. This behaviour may be repeated many times as tests are readministered. It is clear, watching this behaviour, that at least some of the subjects know that they can't do the task and the types of errors made confirm that they can't decide between the two reverse roles. For some reason they can't assign theta roles, or maybe 'map' between the syntactic structures and the theta roles in these non-canonical sentences. Access to the full lexical knowledge of NPs does seem to vary according to the syntax of the sentence. The higher the computational load exerted by syntax, the more likely the fluent aphasic listener is to make errors in thematic role assignment.

There are various factors influencing comprehension in fluent aphasia. A number of factors affect comprehension: lexical factors, in terms of word class, syntactic factors, in terms of sentence type, and grammatical operations. Movement of NPs is a further factor. When NPs are moved from their canonical position, theta-role assignment is less secure. If lexical semantics alone are insufficient to access meaning, then comprehension suffers. The underlying causes of comprehension difficulties involve various domains of language, including syntax. Complex syntax impacts on comprehension at least in the ability to process arguments and their thematic roles within a sentence. If these listeners have poor access to the full representation of verb arguments, this too could impact on comprehension of complex sentences. We also know that factors of frequency and familiarity impact on the understanding of single words as do non-linguistic factors of attention and working memory and maybe mode of input. There is no evidence that fluent aphasic speakers have a damaged grammar per se and there is no case to make here that trace, or the ability to co-index moved sentence constituents, is absent. However, it does seem that sentence complexity, including order of arguments, contributes to the comprehension problems found in fluent aphasia.

Summary

We have reviewed some aspects of comprehension from two vantage points. Firstly, I have tried to convey the difficulties this disorder creates for those who have it and for the friends and families of those people. Secondly, I have reviewed some of the findings from studies of fluent aphasia, concentrating on verbs and sentence comprehension where, in my view, there is still much work to be done. Keeping within this focus, I have summarised some findings from the work at Reading that have led me to believe that, although the grammar is not damaged in fluent aphasia, difficulty with comprehension patterns along predicted grammatical fault lines. In the final chapter I will endeavour to bring the various strands together.

7 *The manifestation of fluent aphasia in one speaker*

Introduction

Although descriptions of fluent aphasia vary, as we have seen, there is one characteristic that is generally agreed to be central, a lexical, semantic deficit. Speakers with fluent aphasia show confusion in their word selection and they have problems with comprehending individual words, and this is thought to be the main reason for their failure to comprehend spoken and written language. Equally, even a casual examination of fluent aphasic speech reveals that production is seriously hampered by lexical errors and word-finding difficulties. The lexical deficit alone, however, will not account for all the problems manifested, and we have considered reports by Butterworth and Howard, Niemi, Goodglass, Christiansen and Gallagher, Caplan and Luzzatti and their research teams, by Blumstein and hers and, in the previous chapter, work by Edwards and Bastiaanse. All these studies have revealed that we can find evidence of grammatical errors in fluent aphasia. In this chapter we will consider data collected from one speaker with fluent aphasia by way of illustrating some of the problems encountered in Wernicke's aphasia. We will examine aspects of his lexical difficulties and consider how far observed difficulties in his continuous speech reflect deficits in syntax as well as in the lexicon. Results from the VAST that have been discussed in chapters 3 and 6 will now be examined in more detail for this subject.

This chapter will start by giving a description of the lexical accessing problems the speaker has in everyday speech and in test situations. It is not easy to locate the locus of damage within the presumed language processes under examination – for example, the processes involved in word production – and conclude that the deficit arises because of problems at point A or point B of that process. Furthermore, not only is it difficult to isolate the locus of damage within the word-production process but it will also become clear that accessing of lexical items is not a process entirely independent of grammar. For example, the grammatical class of a word is associated with ease of access and there are occasional problems with inflectional morphology. The lexical disturbances also disrupt sentence structure but, in addition to this, there is evidence that complex sentences pose special problems. In this speaker, we will observe examples of errors of grammatical morphology, poorly constructed sentences and omission of obligatory verb arguments. We will also view some assessments and briefly discuss the therapy that has been given.

Some background information

The subject to be discussed has already been introduced in earlier chapters. He is a man I am referring to as MG. He has had fluent aphasia for many years which he has borne with considerable fortitude. Despite a severe to moderate language impairment, he has retained much of his pre-morbid personality and interests. He is bright and well informed. He has a good sense of humour, a great love of conversation and debate and has excellent social interaction. He is interested in people, remembers many of the clinical staff he has come into contact with, including students, and, although seldom able to recall names, asks after their progress. Despite his aphasia he has maintained a keen interest in current events, especially politics and sport, and loves to discuss these topics. For MG, who took so much pleasure in conversation and debate, having aphasia has been a considerable burden. Over the years, he has developed a number of coping strategies and a healthy interest in his own language disorder. He has been a willing participant in a variety of investigations as well, attending various blocks of speech and language therapy with qualified staff and students. He always asks for feedback on his performance and, although he has made progress in recovering some of his language skills, he remains critical of his diminished skills and wishes that things could be different, as do we all.

He first became aphasic in 1990 as a result of a stroke while giving a lecture in Cyprus. He was fifty-five. At the time, he was a skilled speaker who frequently spoke in public in connection with his job and as a political activist. A videotape taken of him delivering a lecture at a business conference reveals a confident, amusing public speaker. Not long after the stroke, an initial CT scan was uninformative but a further scan taken seventy-two hours later revealed that there was an infarct in the left middle cerebral artery. The neurological report states that there were changes to the cortex and subcortical white matter over an extensive area particularly in the left temporal lobe and adjacent parietal lobe. At three weeks post-onset his speech and language therapist observed that a global aphasia was present. Comprehension was very limited and his attempts at speaking resulted in jargon with a few intelligible words. (Jargon speech describes output that has normal intonation patterns but few intelligible words. The phonemes used are usually from the language of the speaker and obey the phonotactic rules of that language.) There was a slow improvement over the following weeks and months and within a year or so his profile was that of Wernicke's aphasia. Following the first year post-onset, there was a small reduction in his language deficits and progress has continued over the years. Despite this, his profile has remained that of Wernicke's aphasia, confirmed by testing with the Boston Diagnostic Aphasia Examination (Goodglass and Kaplan 1983) over a number of years and reconfirmed seven years post-onset with the Aachen Aphasia Test (Miller, Willmes and de Bleser 2000). Details are shown below.

Test scores

Some scores from the Boston Diagnostic Aphasia Examination, taken over a number of years, are shown in table 7.1. In these tests, the *word discrimination* and the *body-part identification* tests are closest to what we might consider to be tests of single-word comprehension. In the *word discrimination* sub-test the subject has to select a picture from an array. The arrays are of objects, actions, colours, numbers, letters and geometric shapes. There are six items for each type. Therefore, if we ignore letter, numbers and geometric shapes, this sub-test only tests the ability to recall six nouns and six verbs. Identification of body-parts requires the subject to touch his *shoulder, chest,* etc. The sub-test *commands* is scored according to how many parts of the instruction are obeyed and might also be considered, therefore, as testing the understanding of single words. So, for example, the last and most complex command *tap each shoulder twice* with *two fingers keeping your eyes shut* can gain five points, one for every element underlined. This test does, though, test other aspects of language, such as the listener's understanding of the meaning of other words within the sentences *with* or *keeping*. In addition, the listener needs to understand that the commands need to be obeyed in order. This kind of command also taps auditory memory. These aspects are not considered in the scoring protocol although of course the examiner may note aspects of the subject's performance. The amount of data collected in this test of comprehension is very limited, as we discussed in chapter 4, and therefore limits its usefulness as a means of calibrating a patient's improvement over time. Nevertheless, some change can be observed in MG's performances.

Unfortunately, the results of this test, given in this manner, do not reflect a consistent pattern of performance or even a steady improvement in all areas. Whereas scores for *body-part identification, commands* and *complex ideational*

Table 7.1 *Boston Diagnostic Aphasic Examination: scores as percentiles*
First testing: 30/7/90; Second testing —/10/90; Third testing —/1/91 Fourth testing —/5/93; Fifth testing —/10/94; Sixth testing —/12/96

		1st	2nd	3rd	4th	5th	6th
	Auditory comprehension:						
	Word discrimination	60	60	62	30	65	40
	Body-part identification	45	45	80	80	—	50
	Commands	20	70	65	30	65	70
	Complex ideational material	40	50	50	50	60	60
Naming:							
	Responsive naming	33	60	50	26	83	56
	Confrontational naming	2	49	65	84	83	81
	Animal naming			90	90	90	90
Oral reading:							
	Word reading	60	80	72	65	80	90
	Oral sentence reading	40	80	—	85	83	85
Repetition:							
	Repetition of words	40	90	90	90	90	70
	High probability	52	30	55	65	50	60
	Low probability	40	40	40	40	70	50
Reading comprehension:							
	Symbol discrimination	70	70	—	70	70	70
	Word recognition	80	40	—	60	90	50
	Comprehension of oral spelling	40	30	—	40	60	30
	Word picture matching	60	80	—	60	80	80
	Reading sentences and paragraphs	60	60	—	20	—	70

material would seem to have improved (if we ignore the third testing for *body-part discrimination* and the second *testing for commands*), *word discrimination* hasn't. All scores for these parts of the test demonstrate that a comprehension deficit persists, six years after onset of aphasia, but they also demonstrate that improvement can continue over a number of years and that this improvement can be revealed by standard tests. The scores for naming are also puzzling, while those for reading show a progressive reduction of his acquired dyslexia. The variation of these results is disappointing for a standardised test. However, it is fair to reveal that the assessments were given by different clinicians, in different clinics, over a period of about six years and perhaps illustrate a lack of reliability of the testers rather than lack of reliability of the assessment when given in this manner. An alternative interpretation would be that the performance of the subject varies. Variation in performance may arise as a result of physiological factors or factors related to the individual's life experiences. Cerebral insult can result in long-lasting general effects such as fluctuating energy levels, depression and reduced concentration. These other non-linguistic factors arising from the original CVA may have played a part in the varied performance we have recorded. If that were the case, one would expect to see all scores depressed at a particular time rather than the uneven profiles shown below. Performance may also be related to whether or not the individual is receiving speech and language therapy at the time or to the ups and downs of life such as coping with an elderly relative or moving house. Tested on the Aachen Aphasia Test, seven and half years post-onset, he obtained the following scores confirming the persistence of the comprehension deficit and classification of Wernicke's aphasia.

Aachen Aphasia Test Scores: −9/97

➤	Repetition:	115/150
➤	Naming:	81/120
➤	Auditory comprehension:	47/60
	Words	25/30
	Sentences	22/30

These scores give only a partial picture of MG's problems, and in this chapter samples of speech as well as test scores will serve as illustrative examples of his aphasia. It is obvious that he has problems with lexical retrieval and it is to that aspect of his aphasia that we will now turn. We will start by looking at the deficits revealed in his spontaneous, continuous speech and then look at the deficit as revealed by the single-word test paradigm. It will become apparent that his lexical deficit impacts upon his ability to use well-formed sentences, resulting in ill-formed sentences, incomplete sentences, false starts and mazes. At times, the cause of these ill-formed sentences would appear to be straightforwardly the result of problems with lexical accessing, but we will consider whether some of the errors he produces can be described as grammatical errors and as such are features of *paragrammatism*. This will lead to a consideration of whether his grammar, or access to his grammar, is deficient in some way and, if so, which aspects of the grammar are affected.

Lexical accessing problems

There is a general agreement that one of the defining characteristics of Wernicke's aphasia is word-finding difficulties. Speakers with this condition may omit or substitute words, although substitution, rather than omissions, especially of open-class words, is generally considered to be more typical of fluent aphasia, especially of Wernicke's aphasia. In MG's output, when an open-class word is replaced, the substitution may relate to the target word, either semantically (such as *spear* for *arrow*; *love* for *heart*; *sea-horse* for *unicorn*) or phonemically (*black* for *block*; *knot* for *noose*; *canoe* for *igloo*). Additionally, the fluent aphasic speaker may produce non-words, or jargon, when attempting to retrieve a word. Twelve months post-onset of the aphasia, when assessed on the Boston Naming Test, ten of MG's errors were lexical substitutions while for a further eleven targets, jargon was produced. Many of the lexical errors suggested that he had some semantic knowledge of the target word. For example, the target *tree > leaves*; *pencil > pen*; *harp > French horn*; *muzzle > dog*; *hanger > hat*; *unicorn > horse*. The close semantic relationship with the target word can be seen in these examples. Other attempts may produce substitutions which do not seem to be associated either semantically or phonologically with the assumed target word. The attempts are what Davis (2000:116) has termed an 'abstruse neologism' (*sic*), and a non-word is produced. Such errors have been infrequent in MG's speech although they do appear.

In the following example we will see illustrations of what might be described as phonemic as well as lexical substitutions and a possible neologism. The distinction between what has been described in the literature as phonemic versus lexical paraphasic errors is not easy to maintain as a substituted word may resemble the target word phonemically yet also be a real word, possibly unrelated semantically to the target word.

When talking about his difficulties with his speech during the first year post-onset he claimed that:

(1)   *they can do it but I can't [thay] them . . . . it's gone [ray]*

There are a number of errors here but we will first consider the two obvious errors identified by the square brackets. Both these errors could be considered as lexical substitutions as the substituted word in each case sounds like a real word and hence they can be described orthographically. In the first example the paraphasic error is phonemically close to the assumed target word *say*. If *say* is the target, then the substituted paraphasic *thay* has one feature changed; the voiceless alveolar fricative replaces the voiceless interdental fricative and this suggests that this is a phonemic paraphasic error. If, on the other hand, the error is interpreted as a real-word substitution, a lexical paraphasic error, then MG has substituted a pronoun for a verb. In this case, this error involves crossing word class, verb > pronoun.

The second paraphasic error in this example, *ray*, is not so easily categorised. It is in the verb complement slot within the sentence and therefore the target is restricted in terms of word class. The verb could take an AP or PP depending on whether *gone* is to be interpreted as related to the verb *to become* or *to move*. On the other hand, there is a phonemic relationship with the previous paraphasic error in that the vowel is repeated. However, there is no obvious phonemic relationship with any potential target word nor is there any obvious semantic link between *ray* and the topic of conversation. These words, *they* and *ray*, can be considered as non-words in this context. Both are consistent with phonotactic restraints and sound like real words but only one of them is transparently related to a target word and that relationship is phonemic.

We have now considered two errors of the utterance but there are possibly more for, as it stands, it has little meaning. If a reconstruction is made of a possible, realistic target utterance it might look like this: the actual utterance is in italics and the possible target words are in bold and in curved brackets.

(2)   *they* (**I**) *can do* (**speak**) *but I can't /they/* (**say**) *them* (**the right words**) *it's gone /ray/* (**wrong**)

This reconstruction would give the following substitutions:

(3)   (**I**) > *they*:   pronoun > pronoun
(4)   (**speak**) > *do*:   verb > verb
(5)   (**say**) > *they*:   verb > pronoun? phonemic paraphasia?
(6)   (**the right words**) > *them*:   a pronoun without reference
(7)   (**wrong**) > *ray*:   adjective replaced with a jargon/paraphasic error.

Here we see an assortment of error types: in (3) and (4) there is a within-word-class error; (5) and (7) are probably phonemic paraphasic errors if our guess at the target word is correct; in (6) the NP has been reduced to a single pronoun. In (6), as in (3) and (4), specificity is lost as there is no referent for the pronoun in one and no specific meaning conveyed for the verb in the other example. Such errors and reduction in specificity reduce the speaker's ability to convey meaning.

Words may be produced with fairly clear phonemic substitutions, as in the above example, *ray* for *say* or as in *selben* for *seldom*, an error produced in a repetition task. Where one or two phonemes have been substituted, the target may be clear but other substituted words may only have a distant phonemic similarity as in *naught* for *nine* given in the example of spontaneous speech below. In these last two examples, *selben* and *naught*, the target word is only discernible because in the first case the word was produced as part of a repetition task and in the second example the target word becomes clear because of the context of the NP as follows: *the news at naught* where the assumed target is the name of the news programme of the time, the *News at Nine*.

It is not apparent when listening to spontaneous speech whether these errors should be regarded as errors in retrieving the phonological form of the intended word or whether a whole word has been accessed in error. The problem in identifying the target word is reduced in picture-naming tasks although results on these tasks do not necessarily correlate well with spontaneous connected speech. The benefit of such tasks is that types of lexical substitution become much more apparent and we will examine how he performed in some of these below.

In the early days post-onset of the aphasia, MG produced many errors, substituting words, producing words with phonemic paraphasic errors and producing some neologisms. He used few nouns and few specific verbs which, coupled with the neologisms, made him very hard to understand, but as time has passed, the jargon has diminished and his errors are more frequently omissions or substitutions of words although he continues to make a few phonemic paraphasic errors. We will review some of the problems MG has with lexical accessing, starting with problems that are obvious in his spontaneous speech and then reviewing some test results.

Errors in continuous speech

In the following example MG is describing some kind of outing, linked, perhaps, to going to watch his football team, the fortunes of which he followed avidly. Had his interlocutor not known about MG's frequent trips to see the local football team play, it would have been very difficult to guess what he was talking about. The gloss for the following passage is that he was trying to explain how, although he still went to football matches, these outings were different from how they had been prior to his stroke. His response followed the question 'What do you like to do at the weekends?' In the following transcription and henceforth {f} signifies a filled pause (um, er etc.) and (X) an unintelligible syllable or, when more than one X is given, syllables.

(8)   *I go to the {f} the {f} the Spread and they're very . . . they can get about . . . I used to do that . . . he goes about three or four . . . two chaps . . . him and her . . . he has about three or four* (therapist: whiskies?) *no . . . pint*

This would be impossible to understand without considerable contextual and biographical knowledge. He can neither find the word pub nor complete the name of the pub, possibly, the Spread Eagle. He has not given any referents for the pronouns used (i.e. *they, him, her*) and is probably assigning gender incorrectly in his use of her and *chaps*. For this speaker, *chaps* refers only to males. He is unable to say that the people were drinking but uses the non-specific verbs *has* and *get* and he is unable to say what they drank until prompted by the therapist. Then, although achieving a plausible lexical item *pint*, he fails to give the obligatory plural inflection for agreement with *three*.

On another occasion he was asked to say what he had been doing the previous evening. Here he attempts to talk about the television programmes he watched.

(9)   *I think we did see something or other . . . I can say then but I don't know them . . . XX. XX . . . and they had another girl with a little chap . . . XX . . . and then the news . . . the news at nought er time . . . was news . . . XX . . . and then we had nine o'clock news . . . XX . . . XX . . . and then we went to bed*

This is easier to follow despite the stretches of unintelligible jargon because he manages to say *news* and *nine o'clock news*, after his first attempt, *the news at naught*, but he is unable to say what he had watched before the news. Apart from mentioning the news, he is unable to convey any information that would help the listener guess what he might be talking about.

If we look at the lexical errors within the syntactic structures used, a pattern emerges.

(10)   *I go to the Spread . . .*
(11)   *and they're very . . .*
(12)   *he goes about three or four . . .*
(13)   *he has about three or four . . .*

In examples (10)–(13) above, he starts an utterance but is unable to complete it. He fails to complete the compound noun in (10), and the adjectival phrase in (11) and the noun phrases in (12) and (13). It also looks as though there is confusion with pronominals, for if (11), (12) and (13) are repeated attempts at the same target, that is some information about which of his companions drink. The disruption here in sentence structure appears to result from lexical retrieval and involves the lower parts of the syntactic hierarchical structure, as we have seen in our discussion about connected speech. This differs from the claims made for agrammatism (as discussed in chapter 4). However, we need to recall that the lower nodes are completed sometimes, as in (9) above: *and we did see something*; *I don't know them*; *they had another girl*. Thus structure is available, at least some of the time, although the grammatical consequence is that sentences are often incomplete.

These short extracts illustrate the considerable word-finding difficulty MG experiences, how he relies on non-specific nouns (*something or other*) and verbs (*had*) and uses pronouns without adequate referents (*them, they*). In order to gain some kind of quantification of his lexical errors within spontaneous speech, it is necessary to gain a representative sample of spontaneous speech and then compare with non-aphasic speech. Measures such as noun/verb ratio, type/token ratios of various word classes and frequency of lexical errors compared with non-aphasic speech can give some insight into the type and extent of the lexical problem compared with non-aphasic speakers. Alternatively, an analysis may be focused on some kind of error analysis whereby errors are classified and tallied. Such analyses are described and discussed in chapter 4. The advantage of such metrics is that they give some idea of the extent of word-finding difficulties in running speech, but there are also limitations as previously discussed. Compared with non-aphasic speakers, MG has a low type/token ratio for both nouns and verbs, that is he uses fewer different nouns and verbs compared with a non-aphasic speaker, a defining characteristic of fluent aphasia. The blatant paraphasic errors, although disruptive and diminishing his ability to communicate, are not very frequent being between 3 and 4 per cent of all words.

Testing single-word production: nouns

Few clinicians use spontaneous speech data in their diagnostic process but more commonly use various word-finding tests. As we have seen, there is little indication as to what the relationship is between a patient's ability to name line drawings and to access nouns during conversation. Where attempts have been made to look at the relationship, it would appear to be fairly weak (Berndt, Haendiges, Mitchum and Sandson 1997). It may be that there is a closer relationship at the extremes where the patient has either a very severe impairment or a very mild one, but unfortunately such patients are seldom selected as experimental subjects. There is also considerable individual variation: whereas some patients are assisted in lexical accessing when they see the object or picture, others are not. A number of researchers have demonstrated that how a lexical accessing deficit is manifested can vary considerably from patient to patient (e.g. Berndt and colleagues 1997, Breedin and Martin 1996). Nevertheless, clinicians continue to try to quantify some aspects of lexical retrieval problems by administrating single-word tests, and by looking at scores from these sorts

Naming:	July 1990	October 1990	January 1991	August 92
Responsive naming	33%	60%	53%	30%
Confrontational naming	2%	49%	49%	71%

Figure 7.1 *Naming scores (a) BDAE scores in first year post-onset*

of tests, we are able to get some measure of the relative difficulty of lexical accessing for MG.

In the early stages MG had very poor scores on naming tests. For example, on first testing with the BDAE, he scored only 2 per cent in the confrontational naming section but improved over time. Even so, his scores on naming tests where he is required to name a picture continue to demonstrate that he has a persisting problem with lexical access. The slow improvement can be illustrated by examining the results on three such tests: the percentile scores on the BDAE, the scores gained on Section 53 of the PALPA and the score on the Boston Naming Test. All these confrontational naming tests require a patient to name different pictured items. The Boston Naming Test and the sub-test from the PALPA elicit concrete nouns of varying frequencies. The naming section from the BDAE elicits a variety of nouns and a few verbs. It comprises: six black and white line drawings of objects which are a mixture of high-frequency items (e.g. *key*) and low frequency items (e.g. *hammock*); six actions; two geometric shapes; six colours; six letters; and six numbers. Unfortunately, there are no instructions for the latter sub-test involving digits and *1936* could be named in a variety of ways. For example, one nine three six or nineteen thirty-six. The BDAE has a further test where the patient is asked to provide a word in response to a question. Three of the ten questions elicit a verb, by asking about the function of an object (e.g. *What do you do with soap? What do you do with a pencil?*); four questions are designed to elicit nouns by asking questions such as *What do we tell the time with?* and, showing the age of the test, *What do we light a cigarette with?*; two ask for names of colour (e.g. *What colour is coal?*) and one question (*How many things in a dozen?*) calls for a number. It can be seen from the scores in figures 7.1 and 7.2, that overall, MG's, performance on the confrontational naming task showed a steady improvement while his performance on responsive naming is very varied. This might in part be due to inconsistent marking. When asked a question such as *What colour is coal?* a fluent aphasic may give a fairly long response. An absence of specific marking protocol can lead to inconsistent scoring. Scoring for a one-word response as

Naming:	April 1993	October 1994	December 1996
Responsive naming	26%	83%	56%
Confrontational naming	84%	83%	81%

Figure 7.2 *Naming scores (b) BDAE scores in subsequent years*

in the confrontational task is more straightforward. In 1990, three months after his stroke, MG's performance was poor on these tests. He could name only 2 per cent of the pictures and give the correct response to a third of the questions asked. Over the following months his performance improved dramatically and by seven months post-onset he could name half of the pictures and respond to seven of the ten questions. (Scores reflect speed as well as accuracy of response.) This period is classically regarded as the period of spontaneous recovery but may also reflect direct intervention by his speech and language therapists and MG's persistent practice of tasks set during this time. From about 1993, which is three years post-onset, he was performing at roughly the 80 per cent level on the confrontation naming tasks. His scores on the responsive naming task were more varied and are impossible to interpret. As the scoring within these sections of the test reflect speed of response as well as accuracy, it is possible that a slower response (that receives a lower score) may be more accurate. This is the case for the confrontation naming scores of 1993 and 1994.

The increased scores in the first year post-onset were aided, if not entirely explained, by the processes of natural recovery. After this time, recovery does continue, albeit at a much slower pace. This slower recovery might be the explanation of his improved scores although there may be other explanations. One possible explanation is that the improvement might reflect a learning process, that is, that he learnt from going through the test and, possibly, by asking to be corrected when he failed an item. This is highly unlikely as he was not given any overt tuition on the test items, was not given the correct target and, even if he had been, there was no evidence that he could retain this information. Another possible explanation is that the improvement could be the result of increased familiarity with the test, although it is difficult to see how familiarity with the pictures could aid his lexical retrieval. He had little difficulty in recognising the pictures in the Boston Naming Test apart from the usual difficulty British subjects have with *bagel* and *wreath*. Given this, it is far more likely that the improved scores reflect a real improvement, albeit modest, in lexical retrieval. However, he was left with a considerable difficulty in naming

Boston Naming Test: testing shown in months post onset				
11 mths	16 mths	26 mths	36 mths	76 mths
15%	20%	40%	50%	75%

Figure 7.3 *Single-word test scores: Boston Naming Test:% accurate*

pictures or objects and word-retrieval problems persisted in his spontaneous speech.

If we look at scores on another confrontational naming test, the Boston Naming Test, we can see that this too shows improvement over time: figure 7.3. There is a marked frequency effect for MG as his errors increase as the test items reduce in frequency, but despite his marked difficulty with low-frequency words there is a steady improvement. By 1996, that is six years post-onset, he is able to name three-quarters of the objects in this test. The normal range given for adults between 50 and 59 years (the age group nearest in age to MG) is 82–98 per cent. So, although these scores reflect a real improvement in lexical accessing, MG remains with a considerable difficulty which diminishes his ability to communicate, a problem that continues to limit his activities. Nevertheless, he strives to participate in many of his former activities. A similar score (80 per cent) was obtained (at eighty-four months post-onset) on a similar type of naming test, sub-test 53 of the Psycholinguistic Test of Language Processing, and his scores have remained around this level on both the PALPA and the BDAE tests over the subsequent years. Noun retrieval, then, has been characteristically problematic for MG, although there has been improvement that is apparent in his spontaneous speech and his test scores. Does this difficulty extend to verbs?

Lexical accessing problems: verbs

It is generally recognised that it is the agrammatic aphasic speaker who has problems with verb retrieval (e.g. Zingeser and Berndt 1990), although there are reports in the literature of fluent aphasic speakers with this problem (Berndt et al. 1997). Edwards and Bastiaanse have reported on data collected from two groups of fluent aphasic speakers, one English speaking and the other Dutch speaking. Both groups contained speakers who had low type/token ratios (TTRs) for verbs compared with their normal control speakers. These fluent aphasic speakers were able to produce verbs in the correct sentence position, but the number of different lexical verbs produced was low compared with normal speakers. That is, they tend to have reduced diversity. Comparing the number of different types of verbs used by the aphasic and non-aphasic speakers highlighted the difficulty. A verb deficit may be characterised by a difficulty in accessing verbs compared with accessing nouns, as in the Zingeser and Berndt study, or characterised by a difficulty with verbs. An aphasic speaker may not have difficulty with accessing verbs as a grammatical class, that is, the verb slot is normally filled in sentences, but the range of verbs produced is smaller than the range found in non-aphasic speakers. The range of verbs was reduced for our study and for MG.

The aphasia tests used routinely in clinical assessments have not included materials for eliciting verbs and it is only comparatively recently that the attention of clinicians has turned to verb deficits. (Druks and Masterson (2000) have recently produced a useful battery of verbs and nouns which, although not a test, can be used as assessment materials.) The Verb and Sentence Test (VAST) (Bastiaanse, Rispens and Edwards 2002) has a number of sub-tests that can be used to probe a patient's access to verbs and verb inflection. One of the sub-tests in this battery has a set of forty action pictures that a patient is required to name. On this test, ten years post-onset, MG did not score well, retrieving only 55 per cent correctly. This compares poorly with his ability to name objects as tested on the PALPA, the Boston Naming Test and the BDAE where, as we have seen, he scores around 80 per cent. He retains some semantic representation of verbs as he performs well in tasks where he is asked to select a picture. In contrast to his poor score on naming action pictures, he scores 95 per cent on the VAST sub-test where he has to select an action picture from an array of four pictures, thus demonstrating that his comprehension of verbs is considerably better than his ability to produce them in test conditions.

He also has difficulties in producing verbs in spontaneous speech although this is not as obvious as it is in test conditions. Analysis of samples of his spontaneous speech reveals that although he may use verbs as often as normal speakers he has a low diversity of verbs. This can be expressed as a TTR. We would expect a TTR in an adult speaker to be around 0.7 or above while for MG it is 0.3. We have already seen that when MG uses a verb, there is a tendency to use non-specific verbs such as *do* and this contributes to the low lexical diversity. Low verb diversity has been found to be true for other although not all speakers with fluent aphasia (Edwards and Bastiaanse 1998).

Where do lexical accessing problems come from?

There are various reasons why a person with aphasia may not be able to produce a word in a naming test. Visual deficits may result from some types of brain damage and the most common type to accompany fluent aphasia is a visual field deficit. This may hinder the patient's ability to see the test stimuli but can usually be overcome by judicious placing of the test material. A person with aphasia may also have visual agnosia, a condition in which objects can be seen but are not recognised. Typically, a patient will handle an object, say an electric plug, and signify that they realise that they should know what it is but be unable to demonstrate the use. They may, for example, try to comb their hair with it, usually indicating at the same time that they realise that the action is inappropriate but cannot remember how the object should be used. MG had a mild visual field deficit that he compensated for by moving the materials into his field of vision, and there was no indication that he had visual agnosia. His inability to name items or pictures did not arise from any type of visual defect. Why, then, could he not name objects that he clearly recognised?

Semantic representation

Aphasiologists have proposed that deficits in lexical accessing may arise from different underlying conditions. The aphasic speaker may have problems accessing the semantic representation of the required word. The object is visually recognised but the aphasic person cannot give any information about the object. A zero response may result although the patient may indicate that he knows the target. The patient may recognise the object but be aware that he doesn't know, or at least can't access, the target word. A word with an associated meaning may be produced (for example when asked to name *table*, MG responded with *chair*), or there may be what seems to be a random selection with a word being produced that has no obvious connection with the target word, as we have seen above. Errors that are semantically linked are said to indicate that all is not well within the semantic domain: that is, it is hypothesised that the patient has some kind of semantic representation but is unable to activate the exact word. This is exemplified by errors as in the following taken from one of the PALPA sub-tests: *heart* was named as *love*; *chair* as *table*; *toaster* as *toast thing*. The errors indicate that MG has some knowledge of the target word. He accesses a word that is related in meaning and shares some semantic features.

One way of viewing this close semantic link is to use a metaphoric spatial relationship. Nodes representing words are said to be close to those that are semantically close. Diagramatically, these words are shown as being neighbours and those using this model talk about near and distant neighbours. All near neighbours are triggered in the early stages of the lexical search but the non-aphasic speaker is able to suppress all but the target word, unlike the aphasic speaker. For the aphasic speaker, because all near neighbours have the same 'weighting', that is the same degree of excitation, any of the near neighbours may be produced. It is assumed that in normal production, the target word will receive extra 'weighting' and thus be selected in preference to its near neighbours. Aphasic speakers with problems at the level of semantic representation may be able to distinguish between lexical items that are some distance from each other but make errors with near neighbours.

Some aphasic speakers have more problems accessing words with low image-ability compared with words that are highly imageable. This is true for MG and confirmed on a PALPA sub-test. He was able to select written words that were semantically linked. For example, given *coat, jacket, shirt, bench* and *seat*, he was able to show that *coat* and *jacket* have a closer semantic link than any of the other words. However, we would expect that words that are closely related semantically but are non-imageable would be more difficult for him to distinguish than imageable, closely related neighbours. This indeed was found to be so. On a different task, he was more likely to find a closely related word for targets such as *fog, meadow* and *palace*, even though they are low-frequency words, than he was for targets such as *fraud, malice* and *clue*. One explanation is that the first group of words is more imageable than the second, and image-ablity contributes to the strength of mental representation of the word and is therefore easier to retrieve.

If semantic representation is a central component of language then damage or deficits of this component should result in problems understanding and producing words. MG, despite relatively well-preserved comprehension of single words, shows features of a semantic deficit on certain tasks of comprehension when factors such as frequency and imageability are taken into account. MG does well on other tasks that test understanding of single words. He scored at 95 per cent level on a test of understanding lexical verbs where the task was to select one of four pictures to match the target. He also scores well on a similar task when the stimuli are nouns rather than verbs. These scores are good relative to his other performances but are not at the level we might have expected of his pre-morbid performance. Despite success on these tasks, MG exhibits signs that all is not well with his access to semantic representation. This can be demonstrated in two ways.

Firstly, in his speech, he makes lexical errors and some of these errors have a semantic association with the assumed target. This is true for verb targets as it is for noun targets. However, we can only guess at his intended target word and we can get a better grip on this problem when he is tested and the target word is explicit, as given in the examples above. When asked to produce lexical verbs in response to an action picture he may be successful. As has been demonstrated above he is correct around 50 to 60 per cent of the time. When he isn't successful, various types of errors result. He may demonstrate that he has some kind of semantic representation of the target word even though he cannot access the required verb. Half of the incorrect verbs produced contained some semantic relationship to the target and in each case he indicated that he knew that the word he produced was not satisfactory. Here are some examples: *throwing* was produced for the target *heading a ball*; *picking* as *cutting*, and *it's flowering*; *diving* as *swimming*; *skiing* as *sleighing*; *folding* as *papering* and *newspapering*.

When unable to produce the desired target verb he sometimes creates a verb from a semantically related noun. So, for example, given the target *folding*, elicited by a picture of a sheet of paper being folded, he coins the verb *papering*. I am interpreting that response not as a lexical selection error where he has accessed (*wall*)-papering instead of *folding*. Rather, this can be interpreted as an example of his being able to access the relevant noun *paper*, understanding the task requirement, *produce a lexical verb*, and his producing the nearest he can even though this entails a change to the grammatical status of the item accessed. He adds the present participle ending to *paper* and to *newspaper*, the depicted noun, and so produces the required word class, a verb, on each attempt although neither matches the target. Aware that he was unable to produce many of the correct responses, he would not always try to make a verb but would instead name an object in the picture, at the same time making it clear that he understood that this was not the required response. His responses suggest that his need to convey meaning was more compelling than his ability to seek the correct word class. Here are some examples: *filing* produced as *nails*; *parachuting* as *I know what that word is . . . not aeroplane*; *hammering* as *carpentry*; *watering* as *fire thing*; *milking* as *cow but I can't find the word*.

From these examples it can be seen that MG clearly knows a lot about the word he is seeking and is able to reject incorrect items and indicate that his efforts are incorrect. At times there are no substituted words or attempts to produce the correct response and he will indicate that he does not know the item. One factor that emerges from these tests is the effect of the grammatical class of the words being elicited, with verbs being more problematic than nouns. He scores lower for verb recall compared with noun recall: (frequency of the two cohorts is equal). The grammatical status is therefore seen to be important.

Some of his speech and language therapy sessions focused on his partial semantic representation of words. In the early days, he was given practice in thinking about super-ordinate/subordinate relationships, a task he initially found very difficult. Other tasks included thinking about antonyms and synonyms and working with definitions of words. He was also encouraged to circumlocute when unable to provide a word. Frequent practice increased his scores on the weekly tasks: although improved scores on the therapy tasks were not fully maintained, his ability to name objects did improve over time, as we have seen above.

From meaning to word form

It is clear, however, that problems at the semantic level of representation do not fully account for MG's lexical errors. He also has problems with the sounds of words, especially in naming tasks. He makes phonemic paraphasias and may produce phonemically related items in a naming task. Some of the errors made by MG suggest that he has difficulty accessing the phonological form of a word. This can be clearly illustrated by looking at his attempts to imitate words. Scores on the BDAE show that although he is quite successful imitating single words, he has great difficulty imitating words when they are in a sentence. The following errors are taken from the sentence-repetition tasks in the BDAE. Some of these errors may reflect poor auditory processing where there is one feature error, for example *limes > lines*, but his multiple attempts to repeat some target words reflect the struggle he has in producing the correct phonological form: *plump > plum, clump, clunk, clunker, plumpy*, and finally, *plump*: figure 7.4. He appears to know the target, that is to have a mental representation of the phonological form of the target word, because he knows when he has failed and this leads him to make a number of attempts. He also gets close to the target: many of his attempts miss by one feature alveolar/labial as in *lines/limes*. It seems unlikely that his reduced auditory memory can account for these struggles or for the errors he makes in spontaneous speech.

As some of his lexical accessing problems seemed to arise from accessing the phonological form of the word, some phonological therapy was given. Tasks included asking him to listen to two words and making a judgement as to whether they 'sound the same'. He was asked to listen carefully to words and discriminate between those that had the same or a different initial phoneme or the same or a different final consonant. He was given a 'key' word, for example the name of the village he lived in or his wife's name, and then asked to judge whether spoken words he heard started with the same phoneme. He was asked to do similar tasks for production, for example to give all the names

```
near  > mi

heard > reached                    barn     >        farm
        returned
        wost                       limes > lines

        hearding

                                   plump worm > plum cream

speak  >  speaking                 plump  >        plum
                                                   clump
                                                   clunk
blame  >  flame                                          clunke
                                                   plumpy
sweeping  >  skiing                                plump
             swimming

                                   coat  >         court one
```

Figure 7.4 *Errors from the sentence-repetition task: BDAE*

he could think of starting with the same phoneme, or to name objects in certain categories grouping them by the first phoneme. These and a range of similar tasks were given to encourage him to think about the phonological form of words, at least in the therapy exercises. When struggling to retrieve a word, he was encouraged to externalise his available phonological knowledge of a word. He was asked to think about length of the word (*Is it a short or a long word?*); first phoneme (*What sound do you think it might begin with?*); similar sounding words (*Can you think of another word that sounds like it?*). This strategy, plus similar semantic introspection, as outlined above, would sometimes help him achieve the elusive word or enable the listener to guess the word he was seeking.

The influence of word class, grammatical operations and sentence types

An inability to access phonological form accounts for some of his errors in word production. When tested, it can be seen that he can imitate single words, but it is when he is required to repeat sentences that he makes most errors. Is it, then, that the length of material that he has to repeat is affecting his ability to repeat or does the need to construct a sentence interfere with his ability to repeat words?

MG has a diminished short-term memory as measured by the number of objects or digits he could point to on request. A diminished short-term memory may play some part in his difficulty in repetition tasks, although he appears not to forget the words that have to be repeated but to find difficulty in producing the correct phonological form. In these tasks, it appears to be the added resource requirement of repeating a sentence.

We have also seen that word class has a marked effect on the type of word he can produce. Whereas he can produce nouns in a single-word naming test, he has considerably more problems producing verbs in a test which involves naming actions and many of his attempts result in a related noun rather than the target verb. On the other hand, we can see that he demonstrates some knowledge of word class. For example, many of his errors involve words from the same word class. The tendency to use a word from the same grammatical class holds for closed-class words as well as for open. In the examples above, past-tense verbs are replaced by other past-tense verbs and verb participles by other participles. In continuous speech, he is likely to use lexical paraphasias which are within the same class: for example, *the dog is sitting on the woman*: when the picture stimulus require a response such as *the dog is sitting by* (or *with*) *the woman*. Similar errors are made in written tasks. Given sentences where he was required to fill in the missing word where the required words were all closed class, he failed to complete one sentence correctly: figure 7.5. However, all his substitutions were closed-class words. But there were different types of errors. Pronouns were replaced by other pronouns but prepositions were substituted not only for prepositions but also for determiners. His errors suggest that he had some knowledge of the syntactic requirement of the sentence in that his substitutions, on the whole, respect the word-class requirements of the sentential context. In the examples above, prepositions are put in preposition slots and pronouns in pronoun slots. All the pronouns replaced with pronouns have correct number and gender. The error is with case although this is not a prominent error type in his connected speech.

Lexical selection can cross class boundaries. We have seen above that verbs are more difficult for him to access than nouns, and that when he fails to access a verb, he may substitute a noun in naming tasks, adding an *ing* to form a participle. In his speech, too, he may use a noun when unable to produce a verb. On a repetition test there were no significant differences in repeating nouns, verbs, adjectives or what the authors call functors (Kay, Lesser and Coltheart 1992). From this we can deduce that the difficulty in repeating sentences cannot be accounted for by the difficulty with repeating words from particular word classes. We need to look elsewhere for a possible explanation.

> *John put his car **on** the garage.*
>
> *Sam wanted to know the way **of** Reading station.*
>
> *The cat likes hiding **of** the bed*
>
> *I like going to **of** cinema*
>
> *John misses **you** friends very much*
>
> *I asked Sue if she liked John; she said she liked **she** very much*
>
> *The boy was sad because he had broken **he** leg and couldn't play football*
>
> *I don't know if **his** want to go to the match today.*

Figure 7.5 *Errors with prepositions and pronouns in a sentence-completion task*

There are other factors contributing to his repetition difficulties which can usefully be construed as grammatical. We can see from the above examples that his errors sometimes involve inflectional errors. For example, *speak* is repeated as *speaking*; his attempts to repeat *heard* include *reached* and *returned*, both of which have the incorrect stem but correct tense. However, when he achieves the correct stem, he uses an incorrect inflection, *hearding*. It is not possible to tell from this sub-test whether failure to repeat with the correct inflection is a significant problem. After all, he also produces two participles *skiing* and *swimming* for the target *sweeping*.

When tested with material that contrasts repetition of regularly inflected words with repetition of irregular past-tense words and words with derivational morphology, his performance differs strikingly. He was able to repeat thirteen out of the fifteen target irregular forms of past-tense words and plurals (e.g. *geese, shook, sang*) and 14 out of 15 words with derivational morphology (e.g. *stranger, cloudy*). In spite of this success, he was able to repeat only 3 out of the 15 target words which had regular inflections (*curling, cleaned, pays*). (This material is taken from sub-test 11 of the PALPA (Kay, Lesser and Coltheart 1992). Each of the three groups of words within the test has a control set of words. These are matched phonologically to the test words but have no affixations. MG scored 11, 13 and 14 out of 15 for the three control groups of words. Thus this test shows quite clearly that it is the inflection that is causing MG a problem, not his auditory memory. It is also clear that he understood the task as he correctly repeated three of the stimulus words. His responses

rocks	>	rock
canned	>	can
smiled	>	smile
kissed	>	kiss
freed	>	free

Figure 7.6 *Errors in the repetition of regularly inflected words*

demonstrate his problem with inflection as can be seen in the examples in figure 6. So here we find that he can access the word root, with the correct phonological form but cannot inflect the word even though he has been given a model. This difficulty has been noted for non-fluent, agrammatic aphasic speakers and produced as evidence of a grammatical disorder. An assumption has been made that the aphasic speaker can access the lexical word but cannot then perform the grammatical operation required for tense and agreement. In a repetition task involving single words, there are no syntactic restraints and therefore we might assume that this task could be performed by bypassing the inflection processes and repeating the word as though it were a non-word. This he consistently failed to do.

There is some evidence of tense or agreement errors in his spontaneous connected speech, but these do not occur nearly as frequently as these test results predict. The poor intelligibility of much of his speech, especially in the early days of his aphasia, makes detection of errors difficult. However, occasional errors can be found. In the passage about his television viewing, he says:

(15)   *I can't say much . . . but it's marvellous watching . . . I know but I can't say them . . . you see they had Wogan . . . he come yesterday . . .Wogan . . . he came in . . . that is very good . . . that was very good*

On another occasion when trying to explain what he had watched on television, he said:

(16)   *All the water . . . waters . . . means you comes up the thing . . . all the boats*

In the first example there is a tense error and an agreement error *he come yesterday*. The use of an uninflected verb in third-person position is not part of MG's dialect as can be seen by his second attempt, *he came in*. He also corrects *is very good* to *was very good*. So we would seem to have an error of tense and agreement in this example. In the second example, there is again an error in agreement *you comes up* instead of *you come up*. Yet there are plenty of examples of MG using tense and agreement proficiently. So if he can operate tense and agreement, why does he make occasional errors? It is unlikely that there is deficit at Tense, the argument put forward by Grodzinsky and colleagues (see Friedmann and Grodzinsky 1997, Balogh and Grodzinsky 2000, Grodzinsky 2000a and b) to account for aspects of agrammatism. On the whole, inflection is managed correctly but difficulty with tense is exposed in certain tasks and appears from time to time in his spontaneous speech. These errors clearly involve grammatical operations, operations involving Tense and Agreement, and these indicate that he does not have the same facility for manipulating grammatical structures as a non-aphasic speaker has.

The errors on verb inflection evidence some problems with grammar but this problem is clearly intermittent. There are other aspects of his grammar that are problematic. Although he is able to construct sentences, there are many examples where sentence structure breaks down as we have seen above. In the following sample of speech, it can be seen that, although he understands the task, retelling the story of Noah's Ark, he has problems with lexical recall, which includes the recall of pronouns as well as nouns, problems with using tense and problems with sentence construction.

(17)   *Well, I am Noah and I build the ark and we have, what's that . . . he had*
         build the ark . . . I can't say it . . . have building the ark . . . that was . . . oh
         I know . . . he had . . . I can't say it . . . XXX . . . he has two of the . . .
         cats . . . and two of the dogs . . . how much he go . . . you twelve or
         something . . . two of the dog no horses and four no five of the [X] [XXX] five
         of the [house] cows and five six of the what's . . .

Here, there are certainly problems with lexical access but additionally there are problems with tense and agreement, in the IP node of the syntactic tree (or, if adopting the split-INFL hypothesis as discussed in the previous chapter, in the nodes TP and AgrP), as shown in *he had build, have building* and *he go* as well as incomplete sentences *that was . . .* and *you twelve or something*. An analysis of this sample using Text Units has been given in chapter 4.

These errors are not the most obvious in his speech. By and large MG manages to inflect verbs appropriately, although the fact that there are errors are of interest. Further errors can be induced by giving him tasks and here, where he is required to produce inflected forms of a verb, we see that he has considerably more difficulty with finite than with non-finite forms. In a sentence-completion task (taken from The Sentence Completion Test), given to him nine years post-onset, he was able to produce only one correctly inflected verb in ten sentences. For four of the ten sentences he produced the bare stem: instead of the target *the man waters the garden* he produced *the man water the garden*. For three of the ten target sentences, he produced the non-finite form *the man conducting the choir* instead of *the man conducts the choir* or *the man is conducting the choir*. It could be argued that what he is doing is to produce the citation form of the verb. However, if this was a strategy, one might expect him to do this for all or the majority of the sentences. He doesn't. He produces the non-finite *ing* form for only three of the ten targets. He achieves one correct target *skates*. There is also one neologism *skaking* where the target is *cycles*. In the final item, he failed to respond, indicating that he didn't know how to complete the sentence. In contrast to this performance, when given a sentence-completion task where he is required to supply the non-finite form of the verb, he completed the sentences with the correct verb in eight of the ten items. On only one item did he produce the *ing* non-finite form and for one item he produced a semantically related non-finite form *cry* in place of the target verb *crawl*. It was clear during this task that MG understood what was required, and the fact that he could correctly complete a sentence with a non-finite but not a finite verb would suggest that access to the correctly inflected form of the verb is problematic.

Can these errors be seen as part and parcel of the obvious lexical accessing problems we have discussed above? If we recruit the Minimalist view of verb access (Chomsky 1993), we can assume that errors of tense and agreement arise because the incorrect form of the verb is accessed from the lexicon. Under this model, it is claimed that verbs are base generated with their morphology. Thus the verb is accessed with the correct tense morphology; in example (17), we would expect *he had built the ark* not *he had build the ark*. The morphology has to be *checked* and this is done by the functional projections of TP (the tense node), and AGRP (the agreement node), both of which dominate bundles of abstract features. During the course of derivation, the abstract features have to be eliminated, referred to as *feature-checking* (Haegeman 1999). Radford (1997:70) likens the erasing of features to checking items off from a shopping list. If the features are not checked, then the item is said to *crash*, that is the sentence is ill-formed or aborted. In the examples we have looked at above, such as *he had build the ark*, somehow the verb with incorrect features appears in the ill-formed sentence. Thus it would seem that not only has the verb been

accessed with the incorrect tense but the operation of *checking* has not func-
tioned satisfactorily. Some fault in a grammatical operation allows that form
of the verb through. These errors could be seen, therefore, as a failure of some
part of grammatical operation.

Using the ideas from Minimalism as a descriptive framework onto which
we can chart aphasic errors does not imply that the abstract theoretical ideas
of generative linguistics are describing on-line language processes. However,
if the abstract frameworks have anything to say about the mental architecture
of sentence structure, then it seems reasonable that we can also think about
aphasic language in these terms.

These types of errors are not as common in fluent aphasia as they are in non-
fluent aphasia and they are not frequent errors within this speaker. However,
although not frequent, there is increasing evidence that they are widespread
among fluent aphasic speakers, with reports dating back to at least the observations of Martin and Blossom-Stach (1986). What is more often associated
with ill-formed sentences is failure to access a noun or verb, although word-
accessing difficulties are not confined to these word classes. This failure leads
to incomplete sentences such as *that was* or *you twelve or something*, as we
have seen above.

If errors in constructing sentences can be interpreted as the result of lexical
accessing difficulties and if inflectional errors are seen as a failure to access the
correctly inflected verb from the lexicon, it is beginning to look as though all
grammatical errors can be explained by problems in lexical access. We need to
look beyond these examples for some evidence of faulty grammar that cannot
be easily explained by the obvious lexical accessing problem. People with
Wernicke's aphasia, while having some problems with sentence construction,
can, by and large, form simple sentences. However, when we look at their
ability to use syntactically more complex structures we find some evidence
that this is an area of difficulty, and one that cannot be explained by lexical
deficits.

When the spontaneous speech of MG is examined, we find that, as we would
expect for a fluent aphasic speaker and as we have seen above, he can form simple sentences. In fact if we look at the proportion of simple sentences in a section
of continuous speech and compare that with proportions of simple sentences
found in non-aphasic speech, the proportion in MG's speech is within normal
limits. Using the clause, rather than simple sentence, as a unit of analysis, it
was found that MG actually had a higher proportion than non-aphasic speakers, although the total of well-formed clauses was slightly outside the normal
range (Bastiaanse, Edwards and Kiss 1996). The discrepancy arises because he

has fewer subordinate clauses than normal speakers. It is true that, as observed by Butterworth and Howard (1987), fluent aphasic speakers are able to use complex embedded sentences and non-canonical structures such as questions and passive forms, but there is increasing evidence that they do not do this with the same ease that non-aphasic speakers do. Relevant data have already been reviewed in previous chapters.

The reduced ability to produce embedded sentences or subordinate clauses certainly holds true for MG. In a speech sample of thirty-five Text Units, seventeen were clausal but only three of these were subordinate clauses. All of these subordinate clauses were clausal complements following the verbs *said* and *think*. (A more detailed analysis of this sample has been given in chapter 4.) In the main, his discourse is made up of simple sentences, or matrix clauses, single words and short phrases.

(18)   *And they said yes . . .we're writing . . . and so they went the way and she was*
        at at the boy as he was telling it and must said and they went away and come
        on an they round [crup] at a [XX] [XX] and all the sentences wonderfuland
        she brings this lovely p/big back and and like that and then they go into the
        thing and the little [chaplen] say oh good morning thank you very much and
        they went down to the company and they went and they didn't say
        anything . . . ah gone . . . they said and they looked out the road . . . and it
        was a boy that's gone . . . and he rushed down and he co . . . and he's
        got . . . he's had little . . . he's laughed at . . . because he's had a good
        show . . . good . . . blimey . . . I think he did . . . he was a little chap.

This is his attempt to describe a series of pictures. A series of pictures show a couple preparing for a rather grand dinner party, telephoning their friends, preparing food, setting the table, changing, greeting guests and then, as the guests arrive, discovering that the salmon has disappeared from the table. The host rushes out to buy fish and chips while the cat sits beneath the dining table licking his paws. Without this summary, the reader would be hard pressed to understand MG's version.

Nature of language problems

Scores on tests of naming are not specially revealing. To a certain extent they quantify the extent of the word-retrieval problem and allow us to chart improvement. However, the nature of MG's responses and the types of errors made can suggest the underlying nature of the problem. There is an extensive literature covering word-retrieval problems in aphasia that uses some kind of single-word processing model. In this approach, it is assumed that there are stages in production and that semantic and phonological representation can be differentially impaired. Examples have been given where MG seems to know something about the target word as he mimes an associated action. This does not mean that he has some mental representation of the word at that time and indeed his errors where he uses a close semantic associate suggests that he doesn't. A *snail* is not a *slug* nor is a *unicorn* a *sea-horse*, and he often indicates that he is aware that the word produced is not the target word but that it is his best effort. It is also interesting to note that the alternatives given for low-frequency words have themselves low frequency. It is not, then, the case that, being unable to retrieve a target word, he succeeds in a close associate that has a higher frequency. Nor would it seem that frequency factors play much of a part here, although he has more errors on low-frequency words than on high-frequency words.

Thus it appears that there were problems at the level of semantic representation of words. This was borne out by several clinical activities. In the early stages of his rehabilitation programme, he was given tasks where he was required to sort pictures of objects or written names of objects according to close association. He was then required to select a super-ordinate term for the category. This he found difficult. On the other hand, given a list of paired words, he could recognise synonyms if the words were of high frequency (he scored seventeen out of a possible twenty correct, 85 per cent) but was only at chance with low-frequency words, eleven correct out of a possible twenty (55 per cent). Frequency was also a factor when he was faced with a lexical-decision task, a task he found quite easy even in the first year post-onset. In this task he was required to look at lists of words and judge which ones were real words and which ones non-words. All items were controlled for length. In this task, he correctly judged forty-four of the forty-eight (92 per cent) high-frequency items (e.g., *house, nater*) but scored only twenty-nine out of the forty (73 per cent) low-frequency words (e.g. *exaggerationers, categorically*). Of course, frequency is only one factor that has been found to influence word retrieval as we have previously discussed.

The comparatively high scores on these tasks, especially for the high-frequency words, suggest that MG retains a mental representation of a high proportion of words. Is it, then, that he cannot access the phonological form of the word? We have seen that he does make paraphasic errors where the error has some phonological association with the target word. There are also some examples where he produces jargon. On the whole, though, these types of error are not very common. The examples have been found by searching through test data and samples of spontaneous speech. In one sample of 181 words, where MG was being asked about television programmes he had watched, he produced five paraphasic errors where the utterance was a non-word or jargon. That is, 3 per cent of his words were produced as non-words. In two of them *size* and *blai?*, the targets *Cilla* and *blind* were discernible, but *kiosland bluz* was not. This occurred in the following sequence:

(19)   THERAPIST: *what do you think of the weather today*
         MG: *blimming cold in the morning*
         THERAPIST: [XX]
         MG: *it's cold and well . . . no . . . it's not it's . . . it's hotting . . .*
                    melting
         THERAPIST: *what's melting*
         MG: *kosland bluz melting*
         THERAPIST: *right . . . good . . , when did it snow*
         MG: *last night . . . I don't know . . . in the middle of the night*

In (17) the retelling of the story of Noah's Ark (a sample of 175 words), there are seven non-word paraphasic errors. That is, 4 per cent of the words are produced as non-words. Clearly these errors have some effect on meaning, but at such low frequency they cannot provide the bulk of any explanation. What is apparent in his continuous speech is the difficulty with conveying meaning and this is the consequence of various factors such as: the number of incomplete sentences; excessive use of pronominalization; reduced use of subordination; substitution of words; lexical paraphasias affecting nouns and pronouns. It is the combination of all these factors that characterises fluent aphasia. The speech of the subject discussed in this chapter exemplifies this condition.

Summary

For MG, no domain of language is spared. Access to the mental lexicon is the most obvious problem and we have seen that the problems arise because of poor access to the semantic and phonological representation of words. Grammatical word class also affects lexical accessing and he makes more inflection errors than we would expect of a non-aphasic speaker. We have also seen that his ability to use complex sentences is reduced. Thus, even if there is no damage to grammatical representation, we can observe that he no longer executes all grammatical operations (such as *checking*) as proficiently as he would have done pre-morbidly. The grammatical errors and the reduction of grammatical complexity may arise as a consequence of the lexical accessing problems in that the extra cognitive resources now required to retrieve lexical items impact on the ability to perform grammatical operations. The result is aphasic language that has errors at the phonological, lexical, semantic and syntactic levels of language.

8   *Some concluding thoughts*

In the preceding chapters of this monograph, I have described fluent aphasia from various perspectives, trying to keep a balance between the clinician's view and the researcher's. Many researchers only ever meet people with aphasia within their research laboratories or have only paper encounters, relying on written transcripts or test results. I hope this text provides an impression of how aphasia impacts upon a person and a flavour of what it is like to talk with someone who has aphasia. In order to achieve this, I have drawn heavily on data collected from of one individual, MG, who has been aphasic for about ten years. Data collected from the years following his cerebral vascular accident (CVA) have been used to exemplify classical Wernicke's aphasia and, although his aphasia has diminished, he, like many other people with aphasia, has persisting language deficits. We have examined data comprising monologic connected speech, conversational speech, picture descriptions and responses to sentence and single-word tasks. In addition, data from other people with fluent aphasia, including test results, have been used to illustrate aspects of fluent aphasia. I hope they give some insight into the difficulties speakers with fluent aphasia face every day as well as illuminating the nature of this language disorder.

However, in order to gain a better understanding of this most complex disorder, we need to go beyond what we can hear and observe in daily contact or clinical tasks, and thus we have also discussed some seminal empirical work. On-line and off-line experimental approaches to fluent aphasia have been described and results from these studies discussed. We have discussed studies which, while following similar designs, sometimes produce different results and we have considered how far conclusions from experimental studies match those from observational studies and clinical presentations.

Studies differ in motivation. Some aphasiologists strive to explicate the underlying mechanisms of aphasia, the processes involved in producing or understanding speech and how these processes differ in aphasic speakers compared with non-aphasic speakers. Others describe what they see as the abnormal representation of language, or access to those representations, appealing to linguistic concepts. We have reviewed some of the most influential linguistic explanations of agrammatic comprehension and production and discussed how far such explanations go in providing insights into fluent aphasia. In my descriptions and discussions I have tried to show that, despite the fact that fluent aphasia is a relatively small area of research, it encompasses a variety of theoretical, and not so theoretical, views and interpretations. Some views are expressed with great vigour, although all thinking researchers know that, in truth, we only ever have partial knowledge. We are building knowledge of this disorder and it is a slow process with many setbacks, but we are progressing. In this final chapter I will now briefly consider future directions and then attempt to pull the themes of this monograph together.

Future directions

There are two areas where I predict progress will be made in the next stage of understanding aphasia. One of these will involve laboratory-based research, using highly sophisticated technology to investigate the relation between the function and anatomy of the brain and language behaviour. One of the best examples of how knowledge or interpretations of data slip and slide from one position to the other can be found in the developing field of *in vitro* cortico-neural investigation. Until the latter years of the last century, neuro-anatomical data, gained first from autopsy and later from the early imaging studies, seemed to converge on some version of localisation. The location of neural damage was, by and large, associated with different types of aphasia. Fluent aphasias tended to be associated with lesions in the left temporal lobe while damage to the left frontal area was more often than not associated with Broca's aphasia. However, overlapping with these studies and during the early years of the twenty-first century, an increasing variety of techniques have been used to investigate the relationship between smaller, more precisely defined cortical areas and closely specified language tasks in non-aphasic subjects. We now have results from studies investigating reading, which contrast, for example: nouns and verbs; inflectional morphology; sentence structure; semantic relations; phonemic discrimination. We know from these studies that there is variation in the nature of responses between normal subjects, differences in location of neural activation in normal subjects, and that different studies, different subjects or different techniques can produce different results from what, superficially, promise convergent results. But, variation is so wide and the results so varied that it is often difficult to see agreement, and hence progress, in this very complex field. (It has been said that almost any task can produce activation in Broca's area.) But the knowledge base is expanding, and sooner or later we will have to redefine what we think we know about language, the representation of language as an abstract system and the relationship between neural structures and language behaviour.

When we come to look at functional brain imaging studies that have used subjects with aphasia, the picture becomes even more complicated. Tasks that have been used are very limited. There is no way of knowing if the subjects that comprise a group have similar lesions in terms of loci or size. They are unlikely to have identical language deficits or even the same degree of severity of the aphasia. Furthermore, group members are never exactly the same age or at the same time post-onset of aphasia. They have probably had different types and amounts of aphasia therapy or language stimulation post-onset and have certainly had different language skills or use of language pre-morbidly. Currently, we do not know if any of these factors impact on localisation of language skills or performance on any of the language tasks used in the experiments, and, with the exception of age, we know little about how these factors impact on language function or language recovery. We do not know which, if any, of these factors impact on aphasic performance and thus we are in the dark when it comes to assembling a homogeneous experimental group of aphasic participants. Thus, when group results are presented, we have to take them for what they are – a rough indication of neural activity and, maybe, a rough indication of the relationship between function and neural representation.

Techniques used in brain studies also limit the type of task that is possible. For example, at the time of writing, the validity of conducting fMRI studies that require spoken responses is controversial, as the act of speaking can cause slight body movements that interfere with the interpretation of the signal. New techniques dealing with the data will probably be available by the time this is published (developments can be rapid in this field). Information about production is currently based on subjects reporting silent generation of words or sentences. This area of study is at an early stage, is exciting and holds great potential for expanding our knowledge. However, it is important to recognise the current limitations of such studies and to understand that we are in but the early stages of these studies.

The second area where I hope that there will be substantial progress in the expansion of knowledge of aphasia is in specifying, refining and improving aphasia therapy. This will, in simple terms, involve finding out what does and doesn't work and for whom. It is also hoped that improvement in therapy will encompass recognising what is significant to the person who has aphasia as well as recognising statistically significant changes in language behaviour. This is especially likely where the needs of the client or patient become as important to the funders of research as the research questions being asked. Equally, it is important that the research community recognises that aphasia is a language problem, that language is a multi-component complex system and that is necessary to examine small parts of that system to gain knowledge of it, so that eventually that will help clinicians improve communication in aphasic speakers. Aphasia provides a way of testing linguistic theories, such as examining the relationship between certain pronominal forms and their antecedents by looking at the relative difficulty of certain pronouns, for example. Such research does not only address esoteric questions but eventually influences clinical practice. Trying to find out more about access to inflectional morphology, complementizers, auxiliary verbs or complex sentences in aphasia is part of finding out about the limitations of aphasic communication and will, ultimately, provide ways of informing the endeavours of clinicians. There is potential in this field to view 'theoretically' motivated research as being distinct from 'clinical relevant' research but if we are to make true progress, clinicians need to be informed by such studies and funders of research need to understand the importance of theoretically motivated research.

The number of reports on aphasia therapy studies has greatly expanded over the last ten years. Not only is current therapy often motivated by a theoretical stance but it has been shown to be effective. There are now a number of studies that demonstrate that carefully specified therapy can bring about change in language behaviour in certain domains. There is no clear indication to date that the effectiveness of therapy is associated with any one theory. There is no evidence, either, that any one aspect of language is more amenable to therapy than any other. Reports on improvement in various areas, including comprehension and production of nouns and verbs, and sentence production and reading, can be found in the research literature (see Basso 2003 for a review).

There is no evidence that any one type of aphasia is more amenable to therapy than another. Many therapy studies (e.g. those of Schwartz and her colleagues and Thompson and her colleagues) have used agrammatic participants; some other studies (for example Marshall and her colleagues) have included fluent aphasic speakers while a number do not specify the diagnosis of their participants. Using people with fluent aphasia in therapy studies raises the same kinds of problems that are encountered in other research studies. By definition, some fluent aphasic subjects (especially people with Wernicke's aphasia) are likely to have a moderate or severe comprehension problem, the presence of which demands a very careful design if the effect of therapy is not to be lost by poor co-operation from diminished understanding. There is also the problem of achieving informed consent from participants who have severely diminished comprehension. As a consequence, therapy studies often involve subjects with moderate comprehension loss, as MG exhibits, or subjects with anomia and thus more or less intact comprehension, as in the example of JR that follows.

A further problem for the research community is that most therapy studies involve a single participant or a small group of participants. By and large, there is a relationship between size of group and the detail of the therapy reported. An example of a small study is currently in progress at the University of Reading (Edwards 2003, Tucker and Edwards 2003, Edwards, Tucker and McCann 2004). We are looking at the effect of what we call verb therapy in a series of single case studies, working in collaboration with the local health authority and one of their clinicians. To date, the results of three subjects have been reported. Here I will outline the results for one subject. This subject, JR, a 36-year-old man, started twice weekly therapy at seven months post-onset. He had what many would consider to be a mild, residual anomic, that is, a fluent, aphasia. Although he was scoring towards the top end of all tests, he was still very concerned about his difficulty in accessing words and his hesitant speech. At the end of his twelve-week therapy block there was a significant improvement in his ability to produce verbs, the focus of therapy. He also had fewer ungrammatical utterances in his connected speech, his speech was less hesitant and, as a result of feeling more proficient, he was a more confident communicator.

This is an example of research using low-technology procedures that can be replicated in normal clinical practice. However, there are new developments in therapy taking place in research laboratories. What is truly exciting in the field of aphasia therapy is that, in the last few years, there has been an increasing involvement of sophisticated technology in therapy studies. A synergy is developing between two important areas of aphasia research, investigations into brain–language relationships and therapy. There are signs of fusion in some research laboratories where imaging techniques are being used to investigate whether language change that can be demonstrated in off-line tasks can be associated with changes in neural activity. Brain studies are now being used to move beyond the issue of localisation and to explore the relationship between apparent improvement in language skills and changes in neural activity. Furthermore, some of these studies are specifying, very carefully, the details of therapy delivered.

At Northwestern University, USA, Thompson and her colleagues are investigating changes in language behaviour following linguistic-specific therapy. In these series of studies, they are using fMRI to measure change in neural activity before and after therapy. The therapy given in Thompson's laboratory is developed within a framework of generative grammar. Using agrammatic subjects who have restricted ability to formulate sentences, she is training groups of subjects to produce sentences with verbs and verb inflections, complex sentences with complementisers and various sentences involving movement versus no movement. Her work (and there is similar work in a few other laboratories), which marries linguistically motivated therapy with advanced techniques for measuring brain activity, exemplifies a possible future for aphasia research. It also illustrates current limitations. To date, most studies have investigated comprehension, as it is not clear that tasks involving speaking produce reliable fMRI data, as mentioned above. Studies that make claims about generation of words or sentences by non-aphasic speakers have used silent rehearsal or generation and self-reports of the subjects' perception of what they have generated. There are obvious problems with interpreting results from these tasks, and problems are magnified when the subjects are aphasic speakers. Self-report is even more suspect when the subjects have aphasia.

Studies using brain-imaging techniques are complicated and costly and to date have used small groups of subjects. Unfortunately, many in the medical establishments or government departments and charities that are potential funders of aphasia research are not convinced that small-scale studies produce worthwhile data. Wedded to the idea that aphasia is a medical condition, the only worthwhile design is said to be that of a large randomised controlled trial. The National Health Service in the UK recently put out a call for research proposals to investigate the effectiveness of aphasia therapy, stipulating that it must be a randomised control trial.

Such studies are possible, but they are not only complex and, if we are to look at best practice, very costly, but possibly premature. Further, methodology alone does not necessarily constitute good research. Looking at the effect of unspecified, uncontrolled therapy on large groups of subjects with varying deficits tells us nothing about the potential of aphasia therapy. As Pring (2004) points out, the right questions have to be asked. We need to know what kinds of deficits are being treated and what the treatment procedures are. Any aphasia study needs to take into account the complexity of language, the variations of language deficits that constitute aphasia, the variations of cerebral damage that cause aphasia, the importance of detailing therapy, and the difficulties there are in measuring language change. The list could easily be expanded. Pring suggests that investigations into the efficacy of aphasia therapy would most profitably be considered to be at Phase One, that is specifying what types of therapy work with whom.

All this is not to suggest that measuring the effectiveness of aphasia therapy is more complicated than other potential intervention studies but to highlight that calibrating change and judging effectiveness is complex. Further, since aphasia is manifested in complex patterns, it is not a simple matter that can be undertaken by those with a limited understanding of normal language. The situation is somewhat different in the USA where large grants are given to researchers working with quite small groups of patients. In this work, for example, work by Thompson and her associates (see, e.g., Thompson, Shapiro and Roberts 1993; Thompson, Fix, Gitelman, Parrish, Mesulam, 2000), it is not unusual for groups of fewer than twenty participants to be used.

Descriptive frameworks

Striving to specify the nature of aphasic deficits would seem to be an essential first step in the design of aphasia therapy, yet this is not always the prime concern of therapists. Where an effort is made to specify the nature of the disorder, specification has varying degrees of sophistication. It focuses on varying aspects and may or may not use a theoretical model. Commonly, aphasiologists engaged in therapy look at the nature of the output, the surface form of grammar. A description of aphasia may be built up by referring to 'levels' or domains of language. Note is taken of the errors in different levels of linguistic description: lexical errors, syntactic and semantic errors and so on. The locus of the deficit might then be assumed to be at a level of a model of language processing. Examples have been given in previous chapters of how speech data may be quantified in this way and the locus or loci of the deficit identified. We have used this approach to identify errors in samples of fluent aphasic speech. The errors we have described and discussed suggest that, although lexical retrieval problems dominate, there is evidence of problems in phonological representation and assembly and also in certain grammatical operations.

Another type of data that might be used to motivated therapy is that yielded by standardised tests. The most widely used test, the BDAE, while giving a snapshot of oral and written language abilities, can only highlight areas of relative weakness. Further probes are then needed to specify further details of the language deficits. One assessment that is theory-driven is the PALPA. This claims to be especially useful for finding out more about problems with lexical retrieval and can be used to motivate therapy. The PALPA test, as we have seen in previous chapters, is based on a model of single-word production and understanding, which is used in explanations of aphasic deficits, mainly focusing on single-word production and understanding. The VAST, also reviewed in earlier chapters, provides data about verb production, verb comprehension, sentence production and sentence comprehension in fluent aphasia. We will now review the characteristics of fluent aphasia using the data given in earlier chapters.

Characteristics of fluent aphasia

Looking at the characteristics of fluent aphasic production, we have confirmed that lexical retrieval difficulties in fluent aphasia are a prominent feature. Difficulties in producing lexical items can arise at the semantic level of representation (semantic paraphasias occur) or the phonological level (phonological errors occur). Illustrations of both types of errors were exemplified in the data we have examined. We have noted that psycholinguistic features, such as frequency, affect lexical retrieval for some subjects, but there is considerable inter-subject variation for this effect. For example, for the anomic subject, JR, referred to above, there was no frequency effect in his ability to recall or select verbs. We have also found that, although lexical difficulties are pervasive, they do not account for all the differences observed between fluent aphasic speech and non-aphasic speech. To investigate further, additional types of investigation are needed.

Using speech samples, we have noted examples of errors in verb production, verb inflection errors and problems with sentence structure and that the frequency of complex sentences is reduced compared with non-aphasic speech. Unlike Broca's aphasic speech, the fluent aphasic speech we examined tended to show good sentence structure but not consistently so. Mapping our data onto a hierarchical syntactic tree structure, it was found that errors occurred at both the upper nodes and the lower nodes of the tree. This is in contrast with the aphasic sentence fragments found in Broca's aphasia. In Broca's aphasia, the claim is that the higher nodes on the syntactic tree are more vulnerable than the lower. We note that this pattern of vulnerability is not found in fluent aphasia. The data we have examined are inconsistent, with the filling of various nodes varying from one utterance to another or from one time or task to another. What happens is that the fluent aphasic speaker is not always able to retrieve the appropriate lexical item for every filled node. The consequence of this is that there are many incomplete utterances, restarts and reformulations in connected speech. Furthermore, there is an interaction between lexical retrieval and syntactic processing.

The data presented in this monograph are consistent with the claim that syntax or the grammatical sentence structure has not been lost but the operations to parse or produce sentence structure is not reliable in fluent aphasia. It is generally assumed that grammar is intact in fluent aphasia and this is supported by on-line investigations that we have discussed in earlier chapters. Fluent aphasic participants show that while they have an atypical response pattern to verbs with varying argument structures, they show a normal, although slower, pattern of response to reactivation at the site of moved sentence constituents. These results have been taken as evidence that, in fluent aphasia, syntax is intact although access to lexical items may interfere with the production of well-formed sentences. Thus, it is not the grammar per se but lexical retrieval that interferes with sentence structure. This can be only partly true. Recent data suggest that that is not the complete story. The data collected from a group of subjects with Wernicke's aphasia that we studied in chapter 6 demand an additional explanation.

The data collected from two groups of fluent aphasic speakers, one English speaking and one Dutch speaking, revealed a comprehension deficit for sentences that patterns in the same way as that obtained in many studies of Broca's aphasia. Our subjects, both those with Wernicke's aphasia and, to a certain extent, those with anomia, scored significantly higher for comprehension of sentences with canonical order of thematic roles than they did for those with non-canonical order. One explanation given for this pattern of sentence-comprehension deficit in Broca's aphasia is that trace is deleted in it. That is, the syntactic representation that permits the allocation of thematic role to arguments that have been moved from their canonical position is no longer available. The listener with Broca's aphasia is not, therefore, the argument runs, able to assign thematic role and thus makes errors in sentence comprehension, at least in the tasks given. If failure on sentence-comprehension tasks does indeed result from trace deletion, then we would not expect sentences with non-canonical order of thematic roles to be available in the Broca's aphasic speech. The subjects would not be able to construct sentences not having trace. And indeed, that is what is found. People with Broca's aphasia have great difficulty in constructing sentences and rarely, if ever, construct non-canonical sentences. However, this is not true of fluent aphasia. Here we have a different picture.

In fluent aphasia, we have seen that sentence structure is relatively intact. Furthermore, although the frequency of sentences with embedded clauses are reduced compared with the frequency found in non-aphasic speech, the fact that embedding appears at all means that the grammatical operations required to build such sentences must be available, at least some of the time. A different explanation for the pattern of comprehension deficit is therefore required. We saw that the errors that the English fluent aphasic subjects consistently made were reverse-role errors, that is they confused theta roles of agent and theme.

These particular subjects had scored relatively well on the test of comprehension of single verbs and, not unexpectedly, made few lexical errors. These subjects were not able to access the meaning of the sentence reliably since they could not interpret thematic roles, but they responded at chance level.

If we look at the ranking of the scores for single-verb comprehension and sentence-comprehension tasks, we find that there is not a straightforward correspondence between the two sets of scores save for one subject, MF, who has the lowest scores for both tests. For other subjects there is no such concordance. For example, JoH has the lowest score for the test of sentence comprehension but the fourth lowest on the test of single-verb comprehension; DC has one of the lowest scores for single verbs but one of the highest scores for sentence comprehension. Yet all these subjects made more reverse-role than lexical errors in the sentence-comprehension task. Luzzatti has suggested that fluent aphasia includes deficits within the theta-role, characterised either as a deficit of lexical representation or of theta role assignment. Our data tend to support the idea that it is the assignment of thematic role that is insecure rather than a deficit of lexical representation. These participants were reasonably proficient at indicating the meaning of a verb when required to select one of four pictures to match it, suggesting that retrieval of the meaning of verbs was relatively intact. On a sentence-comprehension task, our subjects performed above chance on canonical sentences but at chance (as a group) on non-canonical sentences. The large majority of errors, on all sentence types, suggested that the assignment of thematic roles was compromised in all conditions but the introduction of syntactic complexity compounded the problem. The subjects virtually never chose the lexical distractor, which suggests that deficient lexical representation was not the underlying explanation. The choice of the reverse-role distractor in all sentence conditions suggests that thematic role assignment was unreliable. Furthermore, the clear influence of sentence type demonstrated that the additional processing or parsing demands of the non-canonical sentences exacerbated the problem. This can be interpreted as a problem with non-canonical order of theta roles or a problem with the grammatical operations involved in forming passive and object-cleft sentences.

However, we need to be cautious when interpreting data from tests. We need to take into account the task effect of a test. We have seen how these subjects were better performers on the single-word task than on the sentence task and have suggested that the grammatical operations involved in parsing the sentence might be deficient. We have noted that these same subjects were better on a task involving listening to a spoken sentence and judging whether the NPs in the sentence were acceptable. This task involved making a judgement about thematic roles. Most participants, though not all, were better on this judgement task than they were on the sentence-comprehension task. These results showed us that assignment of thematic role, although not 100 per cent reliable, was available. On the whole, the group we looked at were better at judging whether the verb arguments in a sentence were acceptable, that is, that the sentence was a well-formed sentence, than they were on a task involving matching one of four pictures to a spoken sentence. Both of these tasks involve access to information about verb arguments within a sentence. It seems that information, or access to that information, is not always available to these listeners and that the type of task used for investigation can affect the results. Performance in this listening task also depends on whether the sentence was correct or incorrect.

In output, we have found errors that suggest that access to verb argument is problematic. Examples have been given that suggest that the speaker is not always able to access the lexical and the syntactic information for verb arguments. We have noted how nouns may be used in verb slots; so, instead of producing *the boy is roller skating*, a speaker produced *the boy is a roller skate*; or, instead of *the man is painting*, the sentence *the man . . . is a painting*. These paragrammatic errors suggest it is not so much poor lexical representation, for in these examples the speaker conveys an understanding of the message that needs to be conveyed. What the speaker finds difficult is accessing the lexical item in the correct grammatical form. This characteristic along with errors in inflection and a reduced capacity to produce complex sentences suggests that access or the implementation of grammatical, computational processes is not always readily available in fluent aphasia.

Thus we see that in comprehension and in production the fluent aphasic speaker has an impaired access to the semantic and phonological representation of words and, additionally, impaired access to an intact and robust grammar. Although grammar is not damaged, in that operations and structures are available, availability is no longer immediate, accurate or reliable. Lexical accessing problems can impact upon the ability to construct well-formed sentences but, equally, the demands of syntactic complexity impact on both production and the understanding of sentences. Access to the lexicon is impaired and so is access to the complete and whole grammar. The result is a reduced capacity to communicate in an effective manner and a chronic condition that has a long-lasting effect on the speaker with fluent aphasia as well as on his family and friends.

References

Albert, M. L., Goodglass, H., Helm, N. A., Rubens, A. B. and Alexander, M. P. 1981. *Clinical aspects of dysphasia.* Vienna: Springer-Verlag.

Alexander, M., Naeser, M. and Palumbo, C. 1987. Correlations of subcortical CT lesion sites and aphasia profiles. *Brain* 110, 961–91.

Arabatzi, M. and Edwards, S. 2002. Tense and syntactic processes in agrammatic speech. *Brain and Language* 80, 314–27.

Avrutin, S. 2000. *Wh*-questions in children and Broca's aphasics. In Y. Grodzinsky, L. P. Shapiro and D. A. Swinney (eds.), *Language and brain: representation and processing.* San Diego: Academic Press, 295–312.

Balogh, J. and Grodzinsky, Y. 2000. Levels of linguistic representation in Broca's aphasia: implicitness and referentiality of arguments. In R. Bastiaanse and Y. Grodzinsky (eds.), *Grammatical disorders in aphasia: A neurolinguistic perspective.* London: Whurr.

Basso, A. 2003. *Aphasia and its therapy.* Oxford: Oxford University Press.

Basso, A., Lecours, A.-R., Moraschini, S. and Vanier, M. 1985. Anatomico-clinical correlations of the aphasias as defined through computerized tomography: on exceptions. *Brain and Language* 26, 201–29.

Bastiaanse, R. and Edwards, S. 2000. Word order and finiteness in Dutch and English Broca's and Wernicke's aphasia. *Brain and Language* 79, 72–4.
   2004. Word order and finiteness in Dutch and English Broca's and Wernicke's aphasia. *Brain and Language* 89, 91–107.

Bastiaanse, R., Edwards, S. and Kiss, K. 1996. Fluent aphasia in three language: aspects of spontaneous speech. *Aphasiology* 10, 561–75.

Bastiaanse, R., Edwards, S., Maas, E. and Rispens, J. 2003. Assessing comprehension and production of verbs and sentences: the Verb and Sentence Test (VAST). *Aphasiology* 17, 49–73.

Bastiaanse, R., Edwards, S. and Rispens, J. 2002. *The verb and sentence test.* Bury St Edmonds: Thames Valley Test Company.

Bastiaanse, R., Maas, E. and Rispens, J. 2000. *De Wwerkwoorden-en ZinnenTest (WEZT).* Lisse: Swets and Zeitlinger.

Bastiaanse, R. and Van Zonnenfeld, R. 1998. On the relation between verb position in Dutch agrammatic aphasics. *Brain and Language* 64, 165–81.

Benson, D. 1967. Fluency in aphasia: correlation with radio-active scan localization. *Cortex* 3, 373–94.

Benson, F. and Ardila, A. 1996. *Aphasia: a clinical perspective.* New York: Oxford University Press.

Benton, A. and Joynt, R. 1960. Early descriptions of aphasia. *Archives of Neurology and Psychiatry* 3, 205–22.

Beretta, A. 2001. Linear and structured accounts of theta-role assignment in agrammatic aphasia. *Aphasiology* 15, 515–31.

Beretta, A., Campbell, C., Carr, T., Huang, J., Schmitt, L., Christianson, K. and Cao, Y. 2003. An ER-fMRI investigation of morphological inflection in German reveals that the brain makes a distinction between regular and irregular forms. *Brain and Language* 85, 67–92.

Berndt, R., Haendiges, A., Mitchum, C. and Sandson, J. 1997. Verb retrieval in aphasia: characterising single word impairment. *Brain and Language* 56, 68–106.

Berndt, R., Mitchum, C. and Haendiges, A. 1996. Comprehension of reversible sentences in 'agrammatism': a meta-analysis. *Cognition* 58, 289–308.

Bird, H. and Franklin, S. 1996. Cinderella revisited: a comparison of fluent and non-fluent aphasic speech. *Journal of Neurolinguistics* 9, 187–206.

Bishop, D. 1982. *Test for the reception of grammar.* Published by the author, University of Manchester.

  2003. *The test for the reception of grammar TROG* version 2. London: Psychological Co.

Blanken, G., Dittmann, J., Grimm, H., Marshall J. and Wallesch, C. (eds.) 1993. *Linguistic disorders and pathologies.* Berlin: de Gruyter.

Blumstein, S., Byma, G., Kurowski, K., Hourihan, J., Brown, T. and Hutchinson, A. 1998. On-line processing of filler gap constructions in aphasia. *Brain and Language* 61, 149–68.

Blumstein, S., Katz, B., Goodglass, H., Shrier, R. and Dworsky, B. 1985. The effects of slowed speech on auditory comprehension in aphasia. *Brain and Language* 24, 266–83.

Bock, K. and Levelt, W. 1994. Language production: grammatical encoding. In M. A. Gersbacher (ed.), *Handbook of psycholinguistics.* San Diego, CA: Academic Press.

Breedin, S. and Martin, R. 1996. Patterns of verb impairment in aphasia: an analysis of four cases. *Cognitive Neuropsychology* 13, 51–91.

Brookshire, R. and Nicholas, L. 1994. Speech samples size and test-rest stability of connected speech measures of adults with aphasia. *Journal of Speech and Hearing Research* 37, 399–407.

Buckingham, H. 1986. The scan-copier mechanism and the positional level of language production: evidence from phonemic paraphasia. *Cognitive Science* 10, 195–217.

Butterworth, B. and Howard, D. 1987. Paragrammatism *Cognition* 26, 1–37.

Butterworth, B., Panzeri, M., Semenza, C. and Ferreri, T. 1990. Paragrammatism: a longitudinal study of an Italian patient. *Language and Cognitive Processes* 5, 115–40.

Byng, S., Kay, J., Edmonson, A. and Scott, C. 1990. Aphasia tests reconsidered. *Aphasiology* 4, 67–91.

Caplan, D. 2000. Positron emission tomographic studies of syntactic processing. In Y. Grodzinsky, L. Shapiro and D. Swinney (eds.), *Language and the Brain*. San Diego: Academic Press.

 2004. The neuro in cognitive neuropsychology. *Cognitive Neuropsychology* 21, 17–20.

Caplan, D., Waters, G. and Hildebrandt, N. 1997. Determinants of sentence comprehension in aphasic patients in a sentence-picture matching task. *Journal of Speech, Language and Hearing Research* 40, 543–55.

Caramazza, A. and Miceli, G. 1991. Selective impairment of theta role assignment in sentence processing. *Brain and Language* 41, 402–36.

Caramazza, A. and Zurif, E. 1976. Dissociation of algorithmic and heuristic processes in language comprehension: evidence from aphasia. *Brain and Language* 3, 572–82.

Chomsky, N. 1988. *Language and the problems of knowledge*. Cambridge, MA: MIT, Press.

 1993. A minimalist program for linguistic theory. In K. Hale and S. J. Keyser (eds.), *The view from the building 20*. Cambridge, MA: MIT Press.

 2000. *New horizons in the study of mind and language*. Cambridge: Cambridge University Press.

Clashen, H. 1999. Lexical entries and rules of language: a multidisciplinary study of German inflection. *Behavioral and Brain Sciences* 22, 991–1006.

Cook, V. and Newson, M. 1996. *Chomsky's Universal Grammar*. Oxford: Blackwell.

Crain, S., Ni, W. and Shankweiler, D. 2001. Grammatism. *Brain and Language* 77, 294–304.

Crary, M., Wertz, R. and Deal, J. 1992. Classifying aphasia: cluster analysis of the Western Aphasia Battery and the Boston Diagnostic Aphasia Examination results. *Aphasiology* 6, 29–36.

Crystal, D., Fletcher, P. and Garman, M. 1976. *The grammatical analysis of language disorders*. 2nd edn. London: Cole and Whurr.

 1989. *The grammatical analysis of language disability*. 2nd edn. London: Cole and Whurr.

Damasio, A. 1981. The nature of aphasia: signs and syndromes. In M. T. Sarno (ed.), *Acquired aphasia*. New York: Academic Press.

Damasio, A. and Tranel, D. 1993. Nouns and verbs are retrieved with differently distributed neural systems. *Proceedings of the National Academy of Sciences USA* 90, 4957–60.

Davidoff, J. and Masterson, J. 1996. The development of picture naming: differences between verbs and nouns. *Journal of Neurolinguistics* 9, 69–83.

Davis, G. A. 2000. *Aphasiology: disorders and clinical practice*. Boston: Allyn and Bacon.

De Bleser, R. 1987. From agrammatism to paragrammatism: German aphasiological traditions and grammatical disturbances. *Cognitive Neuropsychology* 4, 187–256.

 1988. Localisation of aphasia: science or fiction? In G. Denes, C. Semenza and P. Bisiacchi (eds.), *Perspectives on cognitive neuropsychology*. Hove: Erlbaum.

Demonet, J., Fiez, J., Paulesu, E., Petersen, S. and Zatorre, R. 1996. PET studies of phonological processing: a critical reply to Poeppel. *Brain and Language* 55, 352–79.

Druks, J. and Masterson, J. 2000. *Object and Action Naming Battery*. Hove: Psychology Press.

Druks, J. and Marshall, John. 1995. When passives are easier than actives: two case studies of aphasic comprehension. *Cognition* 55, 311–31.

Dunn, L., Dunn, L., Wetton, C. and Burley, J. 1997. *The British Picture Vocabulary Scales*. Windsor: NFER-Nelson.

Edwards, S. 1995. Profiling fluent aphasic spontaneous speech: a comparison of two methodologies. *European Journal of Disorders of Communication* 30, 333–45.

   2000. Grammar and fluent aphasia. *Brain and Language* 74, 560–63.

   2003. Aphasia therapy. Paper given at fourth Science of Aphasia Conference, Trieste, Italy.

Edwards, S. and Bastiaanse, R. 1998. Diversity in the lexical and syntactic abilities of fluent aphasic speakers. *Aphasiology* 12, 99–117.

Edwards, S. and Garman, M. 1989. Case study of a fluent aphasic: the relationship between linguistic assessment and therapeutic intervention. In P. Grunwell and A. James (eds.). *The functional evaluation of language disorders*. London: Croom Helm.

Edwards, S., Garman, M. and Knott, R. 1995. Grammatical analysis of aphasic speech: the potential of unmarked sources of evidence. *Brain and Language* 51, 103–6.

Edwards, S. and Knott, R. 1994. Assessing spontaneous language abilities of aphasic speakers. *Testing* 11, 49–64.

Edwards, S. and Salis, C. (in press). Adaptation theory and non-fluent aphasia in English speakers. *Aphasiology*.

Edwards, S., Tucker, K. and McCann, C. 2004. The contribution of verb retrieval to sentence construction: a clinical study. *Brain and Language* 91, 78–9.

Eggert, G. (ed.). 1977. *Wernicke's works on aphasia*. The Hague: Mouton.

Ellis, A. and Young, A. 1988. *Human cognitive neuropsychology*. London: Erlbaum.

Francis, W. and Kucera, H. 1982. *Frequency analysis of English language usage: lexicon and grammar*. Boston, MA: Houghton Miflin.

Friedmann, N. 2000. Moving verbs in agrammatic production. In R. Bastiaanse and Y. Grodzinsky (eds.), *Grammatical disorders in aphasia*. London: Whurr.

Friedmann, N. and Grodzinsky, Y. 1997. Verb inflection in agrammatism: pruning the syntactic tree. *Brain and Language* 56, 397–425.

Garman M. 1989. The role of linguistics in speech therapy: assessment and interpretation. In P. Grunwell and A. James (eds.), *The functional evaluation of language disorders*. London: Croom Helm.

Garman, M. and Edwards, S. 1995. Syntactic assessment of expressive language. In K. Grundy (ed.), *Linguistics in clinical practice*. 2nd edn. London: Taylor and Francis.

Garrett, M. F. 1975. The analysis of sentence production. In G. Bower (ed.), *The psychology of learning and motivation*. New York: Academic Press.

   1976. Syntactic processes in sentence production. In R. J. Wales and E. Walker (eds.), *New approaches to language mechanisms*. Amsterdam: Holland.

   1988. Processes in language production. In F. J. Newmyer (ed.), *Linguistics: the Cambridge survey. Vol. III: Language: psychological and biological aspects*. Cambridge: Cambridge University Press.

Gerschwind, N. 1966. Carl Wernicke, the Breslau School and the history of aphasia. In E. C. Carterette (ed.), *Brain function III speech, language and communication.* Berkeley: University of California Press.

Gleason, J. B., Goodglass, H., Obler, L., Green, E., Hyde, M. and Weintraub, S. 1980. Narrative strategies of aphasic and normal-speaking subjects. *Journal of Speech and Hearing Research* 23, 370–82.

Goldman, R., Schwartz, M. and Wiltshire, C. 2001. The influence of phonological context on the sound errors a speaker makes. *Brain and Language* 78, 279–307.

Goodglass, H. 1993. *Understanding aphasia.* San Diego: Academic Press.

Goodglass, H., Christiansen, J. and Gallagher, R. 1993. Comparison of morphology and syntax in free narrative and structured tests: fluent vs. non-fluent aphasics. *Cortex* 29, 131–405.

Goodglass, H. and Hunt, J. 1958. Grammatical complexity and aphasic speech. *Word* 14, 197–207.

Goodglass, H. and Kaplan, E. 1972. *The assessment of aphasia and related disorders.* Philadelphia: Lea and Febiger.

   1983. *The assessment of aphasia and related disorders.* 2nd edn. Philadelphia: Lea and Febiger.

Goodglass, H., Kaplan, E. and Barresi, B. 2001. *The assessment of aphasia and related disorders.* 3rd edn. London: Lippincott Williams and Wilkins.

Goodglass, H., Kaplan, E. and Weintraub, S. 1983. *The Boston Naming Test.* Philadelphia: Lea and Febiger.

Goodglass, H., Quadfasel, F. A. and Timberlake, W. H. 1964. Phrase length and the type and severity of aphasia. *Cortex* 1, 133–53.

Grodzinsky, Y. 1990. *Theoretical perspectives on language deficits.* Cambridge, MA: MIT Press.

   1991. There is an entity called agrammatism. *Brain and Language* 41, 555–64.

   1995. A restrictive theory of agrammatic comprehension. *Brain and Language* 50, 27–51.

   1995. Trace deletion, theta roles and cognitive strategies. *Brain and Language* 51, 469–97.

   2000a. The neurology of syntax: language without Broca's area. *Behavioral and Brain Sciences* 23, 1–32.

   2000b. Overarching agrammatism. In Y. Grodzinsky, L. Shapiro and D. Swinney (eds.), *Language and the Brain: representation and processing.* San Diego: Academic Press.

Haegeman, L. 1994. *Government and Binding Theory.* 2nd edn. Oxford: Blackwell.

Hagiwara, H. 1993. The breakdown of Japanese passives and theta-role assignment principle by Broca's aphasics. *Brain and Language* 45, 318–39.

   1995. The breakdown of functional categories and the economy of derivation. *Brain and Language* 50, 92–117.

Hagoort, P., Brown, C. and Osterhout, L. 1999. The neurocognition of syntactic processing. In C. Brown and P. Hagoort (eds.), *The neurocognition of language.* Oxford: Oxford University Press.

Hagoort, P. and Kutas, M. 1995. Electrophysiological insights into language deficits. In F. Boller and J. Grafman (eds.), *Handbook of Neuropsychology,* Vol. X.

Hagoort, P., Wassenaar, M. and Brown, C. 2003. Syntax-related ERP-effects in Dutch. *Cognitive Brain Research* 16, 38–50.

Harley, T. 1995. *The psychology of language.* Hove: Psychology Press.

Harley, T. 2004. Does cognitive psychology have a future? *Cognitive Neuropsychology* 21, 3–16.

Head, Henry. 1920. Aphasia: an historical review. *Proceedings of the Society of Neurology of the Royal Society of Medicine*, 390–411.

Hesketh, A. and Bishop, D. 1996. Agrammatism and adaptation theory. *Aphasiology* 10, 49–80.

Hickok, G. 1992. *Agrammatic comprehension and trace deletion hypothesis.* Occasional Paper No. 45, MIT Centre for Cognitive Science.

1993. Parallel parsing: evidence from re-activation in garden-path sentences. *Journal of psycholinguistic Research* 22, 239–50.

Hickok, G. and Avrutin, S. 1996. Representation, referentiality and processing in agrammatic comprehension: two case studies. *Brain and Language* 50, 10–26.

1996. *Wh*-questions in two Broca's aphasiacs. *Brain and Language* 52, 314–27.

Hollis, A. 2002. New techniques for identifying the neural substrate of language and language impairments. *Aphasiology* 16, 855–7.

Hollis, A. and Heidler, J. 2002. Mechanism of early aphasia recovery. *Aphasiology* 16, 885–95.

Howard, D. 1997. Language in the human brain. In M. Rugg (ed.), *Cognitive neuropsychology.* Hove: Psychology Press.

Howes, D. 1964. Application of the word-frequency concept to aphasia. In A. V. de Reuck and M. O'Connor (eds.), *Disorders of language.* London: Churchill.

Howes, D. and Gerschwind, N. 1964. Quantitative studies of aphasic language. *Ass. Res. Nerv. Ment. Dis.* 42, 229–44.

Huber, W., Poeck, K., Weniger, D. and Willmes, K. 1983. *The Aachen Aphasia Test.* Goettingen: Hogrefe.

Huber, W., Poeck, K. and Willmes, K. 1984. The Aachen Aphasia Test (AAT). *Advances in Neurology* 42, 291–303.

Inglis, A. L. 2003. Taking expectations to task in aphasic sentence comprehension: investigations of off-line performance. *Aphasiology* 17, 265–89.

Jain, B. 2004. Model based intervention for sentence production disorders in patients with aphasia. Unpublished doctoral dissertation. University of Canterbury, New Zealand.

Jaeger, J. J., Lockwood, A. H., Kemmerer, D. L., van Valin, R. D., Murphy, B. W. and Khalak, H. G. 1996. A positron emission tomographic study of regular and irregular verb morphology in English. *Language* 72, 451–97.

Just, M. and Carpenter, P. 1992. A capacity theory of comprehension: Individual differences in working memory. *Psychological Review* 99, 122–49.

Kay, J., Lesser, R. and Coltheart, A. 1992. *The psycholinguistic analysis of language processing.* Hove: Psychology Press.

Kertesz, A. 1982. *The Western Aphasia Battery.* New York: Grune and Statton.

Kolk, H. and Heeschen, C. 1992. Agrammatism, paragrammatism and the management of language. *Language and Cognitive Processes* 7, 89–129.

Lesser, R. 1978. *Linguistics aspects of aphasia.* London: Arnold.

Levelt, W. 1989. *Speaking: from intention to articulation.* Cambridge, MA: MIT Press.

Levelt, W., Roelofs, A. and Meyer, A. 1999. A theory of lexical access in speech production. *Behavioral and Brain Sciences* 22, 1–75.

Lichtheim, L. 1885. On aphasia. *Brain* 7, 433–83.

Luzzatti, C., Raggi, R., Zonca, G., Pistarni, C., Contardi, A. and Pinna, G. 2002. On the nature of selective impairment of verb and noun retrieval. *Cortex* 37, 724–6.

Luzzatti, C., Toraldo, A., Guasti, M., Ghirardi, G., Lorenzi, L. and Guarnaschelli, C. 2001. Comprehension of reversible active and passive sentences in agrammatism. *Aphasiology* 15, 419–41.

Marshall, John. 1995. Acquired disorders of language: from Gesner to Goodglass (and back again). Review: *Understanding Aphasia* by H. Goodglass. *Language and Speech* 38, 307–10.

Marshall, Jane, Black, M., Byng, S., Chiat, S. and Pring, T. (eds.) 1999. The sentence processing resource pack. Oxon: Winslow Press.

Marshall, Jane, Chiat, S. and Pring, T. 1997. An impairment in processing verbs' thematic roles: a therapy study. *Aphasiology* 11, 855–76.

Martin, N. and Gupta, P. 2004. Exploring the relationship between word processing and verbal short-term memory: evidence from associations and dissociations. *Cognitive Neuropsychology* 21, 213–28.

Martin, R. 1995. Working memory doesn't work: a critique of Miyake et al.'s Capacity Theory of aphasia comprehension deficits. *Cognitive Neuropsychology* 12, 623–36.

Martin, R. and Blossom-Stach, C. 1986. Evidence of syntactic deficits in a fluent aphasic. *Brain and Language* 28, 196–234.

McCann, C. and Edwards, S. 2002. Verb problems in fluent aphasia. *Brain and Language* 83, 42–4.

  2003. Fractionating the comprehension deficit in fluent aphasia: adding to the data. Paper given at Verb Seminar: University College London.

Miller, N., Willmes, K. and de Bleser, R. 2000. The psychometric properties of the English language version of the Aachen Aphasia Test (EAAT). *Aphasiology* 14, 683–722.

Miyake, A., Carpenter, P. and Just, M. 1994. A capacity approach to syntactic comprehension disorders: making normal adults perform like aphasic patients. *Cognitive Neuropsychology* 11, 671–717.

Niemi, J. 1990. Nonlexical grammatical deviations in 'paragrammatic' aphasia. *Folia Linguistica* 24, 389–404.

Obler, L. and Gjerlow, K. 1999. *Language and the brain.* Cambridge: Cambridge University Press.

Ojemann, G. 1994. Cortical stimulation and recording in language. In A. Kertesz (ed.), *Localisation and neuroimaging in neuropsychology.* New York: Academic Press.

Ouhalla, J. 1993. Functional categories, agrammatism and language acquisition. *Linguistic Berichte* 143, 3–36.

Paulesu, E., Frith, E. and Frackowiak, R. 1993. The neural correlates of the verbal component of working memory. *Nature* 362, 342–5.

Penn, C. 2000. Aphasia in Afrikaans: a preliminary analysis. Paper given at Aphasia Rehabilitation Conference, Rotterdam, The Netherlands.

Pesetsky, D. 1987. *Wh-in-situ: movement and unselective binding.* Cambridge, MA: MIT Press.

Poeck, K. 1989. Fluency. In C. Code (ed.), *The characteristics of aphasia.* Hove: Erlbaum.

Poeppel, D. 1996. A critical review of PET studies of phonological processing. *Brain and Language* 55, 317–51.

Pollock, J. 1989. Verb movement, Universal Grammar, and the structure of IP, *Linguistic Inquiry* 20, 365–424.

Pring, T. 2004. Ask a silly question: two decades of troublesome trials. *International Journal of Language and Communication Disorders* 39, 285–302.

Prins, R., Snow, C. and Wagenaar, E. 1978. Recovery from aphasia: spontaneous speech versus language comprehension. *Brain and Language* 6, 192–211.

Pustejovsky, J. 1995. *The generative lexicon.* Cambridge, MA: MIT Press.

Quirk, R., Greenbaum, S. and Leech, G. 1985. *A comprehensive grammar of the English language.* Harlow: Longman.

Quirk, R., Greenbaum, S., Leech, G. and Svartrik, J. 1972. *A grammar of contemporary English.* London: Longman.

Radford, A. 1997. *Syntax: a Minimalist introduction.* Cambridge: Cambridge University Press.

Rapcsak, S. and Rubens, A. 1994. Localization of lesions in transcortical aphasia. In A. Kertesz (ed.), *Localization and neuroimaging in neuroimaging in neuropsychology.* London: Academic Press.

Rosen, S. T. 1996. Events and verb classification. *Linguistics* 34, 191–223.

Saffran, E., Berndt, R. and Schwartz, M. 1989. The quantitative analysis of agrammatic production: procedures and data. *Brain and Language* 37, 440–79.

Schwartz, M. 1987. Patterns of speech production deficits within and across aphasia syndromes: application of a psycholinguistic model. In M. Coltheart, G. Sartori and R. Job (eds.), *The cognitive neuropsychology of language.* Hove: Lawrence Erlbaum.

Schwartz, M., Saffran, E., Myers, J. and Martin, R. 1994. Mapping therapy: a treatment program for agrammatism. *Aphasiology* 8, 19–54.

Shalice, T. 2004. On Harley on Rapp. *Cognitive Neuropsychology* 21, 41–3.

Shapiro, L. 2000. Some recent investigations of gap filling in normal listeners: implications for normal and disordered language processing. In Y. Grodzinsky, L. Shapiro and D. Swinney (eds.), *Language and the Brain.* San Diego: Academic Press.

Shapiro, L., Gordon, B., Hack, N. and Killackey, J. 1993. Verb-argument structure processing in complex sentences in Broca's and Wernicke's aphasia. *Brain and Language* 45, 423–47.

Shapiro, L. and Levine, B. 1990. Verb processing during sentence comprehension in aphasia. *Brain and Language* 38, 21–47.

Smith, E. and Geva, A. 2000. Verbal working memory and its connections to language processing. In Y. Grodinsky, L. Shapiro and D. Swinney (eds.), *Language and the Brain.* San Diego: Academic Press.

Smith, N. 1999. *Chomsky: ideas and ideals.* Cambridge: Cambridge University Press.

Swaab, T., Brown, C. and Hagoort, P. 1997. Spoken Sentence comprehension in aphasia: event-related potential evidence for a lexical integration deficit. *Journal of Cognitive Neuroscience* 9, 1, 39–66.

Swinney, D., Zurif, E. and Nicol, J. 1989 The effects of focal brain damage on sentence processing: an examination of the neurological organisation of a mental module. *Journal of Cognitive Neuroscience* 1, 25–37.

Swinney, D., Zurif, E., Prather, P. and Love, T. 1996. The neurological distribution of processing operations underlying language comprehension. *Journal of Cognitive Neuroscience* 8, 174–84.

Swinney, D. and Zurif, E. 1995. Syntactic processing in aphasia. *Brain and Language* 50, 225–39.

Thompson, C. K. (in press). Functional neuro-imaging: applications for studying aphasia. In L. L. LaPointe (ed.), *Aphasia and related neurogenic language disorders.* 3rd edn. New York: Thieme.

Thompson, C. K. and Faroqi Shah, Y. 2002. Models of sentence production. In A. Hillis (ed.), *The handbook of adult language disorders.* New York: Psychology Press.

Thompson, C. K., Lange, K., Schneider, S. and Shapiro, L. 1997. Agrammatic and non-brain damaged subjects' verb and argument structure production. *Aphasiology* 11, 473–90.

Thompson, C. K., Fix, S., Gitelman, D., Parrish, T. and Mesulam, M. 2000. FMRI studies of agrammatic sentence comprehension before and after treatment. *Brain and Language* 74, 387–91.

Thompson, C. K. and Shapiro, L. P. 1995. Training sentences in agrammatism: implications for normal and disordered language. *Brain and Language* 50, 201–24.

Thompson, C. K., Shapiro, L., Kiran, S. and Sobecks, J. 2003. The role of syntactic complexity in treatment of sentence deficits in agrammatic aphasia: the complexity account of treatment efficacy (CATE). *Journal of Speech, Language and Hearing Research* 46, 591–607.

Thompson, C. K., Shapiro, L., Li, L. and Schendel, L. 1994. Analysis of verbs and verb argument structure: a method for quantification of agrammatic language production. *Clinical Aphasiology* 23, 121–40.

Thompson, C. K., Shapiro, L. and Roberts, M. 1993. Treatment of sentence production deficits in aphasia: a linguistic-specific approach to *wh*-interrogative training and generalization. *Aphasiology* 7, 111–33.

Tyler, L. K., Bright, P., Fletcher, P. and Stamatakis, E. 2004. Neural processing of nouns and verbs: the role of inflectional morphology. *Neuropsychologia* 42, 512–23.

Tyler, L. K., Russell, R., Fadili, J. and Moss, H. 2001. The neural representation of nouns and verbs: PET studies. *Brain* 124, 1619–34.

Ullman, M., Corkin, S., Coppola, M., Hickok, G. and Koroshetz, W. et al. 1997. A neural dissociation within language: evidence that the mental dictionary is part of declarative memory and that grammatical rules are processed by the procedural system. *Journal of Psycholinguistic Research* 30, 37–69.

Wallesch, C., Bak, T. and Schulle-Monting, J. 1992. Acute aphasia – patterns and prognosis. *Aphasiology* 6, 373–85.

Wepman, J. and Jones, L. 1961. *Language modality test for aphasia*. Chicago: University of Chicago Press.

Wernicke, C. 1874/1977. *Der aphasische symptomencomplex: ein psychologische studie auf anatomische basis*. In G. H. Eggert (ed.), *Wernicke's works on aphasia: a source book and review*. The Hague: Mouton.

Willmes, K. and Poeck, K. 1993. To what extent can aphasic syndromes be localised? *Brain* 116, 1527–40.

Wise, R., Chollet, F., Hadar, U., Friston, K., Hoffner, E. and Frackowiak, R. 1991. Distribution of cortical neural networks involved in word comprehension and word retrieval. *Cortex* 114, 1803–17.

Zingeser, I. and Berndt, R. 1990. Retrieval of nouns and verbs in agrammatism and anomia. *Brain and Language* 39, 14–32.

Zurif, E. 1995. Brain regions of relevance to syntactic processing. In L. Gleitman and M. Liberman (eds.). *Language*. Cambridge: Cambridge University Press.

Zurif, E. and Pinange, M. 2000. Semantic composition: processing parameters and neuroanatomical considerations. In R. Bastiaanse and Y. Godzinsky (eds.), *Grammatical disorders in aphasia: a neurolinguistic perspective*. London: Whurr.

Zurif, E. and Swinney, D. 1994. Neuropsychology of sentence comprehension. In M. A. Gernsbacher (ed.), *Handbook of psycholinguistics*. Orlando, FL: Academic Press.

Zurif, E., Swinney, D., Prather, P., Solomon, J. and Bushell, C. 1993. An on-line analysis of syntactic processing in Broca's aphasia and Wernicke's aphasia. *Brain and Language* 45, 448–64.

Index